I0520769

UPRISE

THE BODY GUITAR THEORY® AND BACK PAIN LIBERATION

SEAN M. WHEELER, MD

UPRISE

THE BODY GUITAR THEORY® AND BACK PAIN LIBERATION

BODY ⟩ GUITAR

2ND EDITION

UPRISE

Copyright ©2015 by Body Guitar LLC
Edition 2 Copyright ©2025 by Body Guitar LLC

All rights reserved, including the right of reproduction in whole or in part in any form.

Body Guitar, Tune Me, Bracing Muscle, Action Muscle, Deep Bracing Muscle, String Muscle, Stability Gap and 180 in 180 are trademarks of Sean M. Wheeler, M.D., for which applications for registration are complete or pending with the US Patent and Trademark Office.

For information contact UPRISE@BodyGuitar.com or visit www.BodyGuitar.com

The reader should consult a physician in matters relating to his/her health, particularly for any symptoms that may require diagnosis or medical attention.

Printed in the United States of America.

Ebook ISBN: 979-8-9935960-0-6
Paperback ISBN: 979-8-2700-7975-8 (Amazon)
979-8-9935960-1-3 (IngramSpark)
Hardcover ISBN: 979-8-2700-8039-6 (Amazon)
979-8-9935960-2-0 (IngramSpark)

Library of Congress Control Number: 2025922588

Cover design, Illustrations and Creative Direction:
Tracy Holdeman & Steve Cranford/WHISPERglobally.com
Second Edition Book Interior:
Suzanne Hurtig/SuzanneHurtigDesign.com

Cover Design, Illustrations and Photography
©2015, 2025 Body Guitar LLC

Second Edition Sean M. Wheeler, MD

TO MY WIFE, SUSIE,

my best friend, my partner, and the love of my life.

CONTENTS

ACKNOWLEDGMENTS

You don't spend years writing a book without some significant help. None of this would have been possible without the help of those around me. I want to thank the doctors, nurses, and people of Belleville, Kansas, who helped me develop my early medical ideas.

To the wonderful staff at The Body Guitar Clinic who have seen us through these early years and continue to plug away as we keep the faith and try to change the world of back and neck pain. Especially Julie Bussell and Demetris Jones, whose belief in me and the clinic is unrivaled. Duke Wheeler, Stacy Madmon-Riester, Amy Barbour, Hannah Garrett, Paige Bowles, Sandra Helton, Toni Atwood, Amber Roderick. Nurse Practitioners Zach Watt, Susanne Conrad, Grace Keltner, Melanie Hijaz and Physician Assistant Rene Heberlie.

To my staff, doctors, and administrators at College Park who put up with me and supported me through all these years, especially Demetris Jones and Leah Van Wyngarden, who supported me and my practice in so many ways; also Sherra Brown, Lindsey Hanna, Kelli Brodie, Dan Kalhman, Samantha Mathias, Shannon Cabera, Lacey

Pierce-Dawson, the late Lonnie Striegal, Stephanie Lee, Laura Van Heimer, Cathy Sims, Brandy Burns, and Tracey Shafer. And my nurse practitioners and physician assistants Grace Keltner, Rene Heberlie, (yes they worked both places) Ashley Fallucca, Mackinzie Maxon, Meghan Kahler, Hanna Wilhette, Shelly Duke, and John Radcliff.

To my partners Dr. Dan Gurley, Dr. Lan Knoff, and Dr. Bob Gibbons, who has listened to my "crazy" ideas for years.

To the people who have helped me with the editing of this book, including Laura Kalhman, Deborah Shouse, Dylan Streeter, and Andrew Mortazavi. Also, Lynne Litt who provided touches that we would be "Lost" without. For my life long friend Barry Maupin who singlehandedly took on editing the second edition and made everything so much better. Jeff Tauscher, David Poulter and Dr. Lynda Prince who provided last minute tweaking.

To the physical therapists who helped me care for my patients and have been sounding boards for my ideas through the years, including Jake Mcfarland, Mike Sabolovic, Carol Higgerson, Brian Adams, Mark Buckingham, Dan Lorenz, Abby Bodenhausen, Teresa Rose, Michael Denning, Derek Fiest, Melissa Church, Hailey Smith, Olivia Smith, Donnie Dequine, Sushma Patel, Sydney Dowding, Max Stonekin and the other therapists of College Park Family Care Center. Especially to Shelley Lewis, who has taught me so much that I sometimes wonder where my part of the book begins, and hers ends. Shelley has been a filter through which so many of my ideas have passed and been transformed and tweaked that I cannot adequately express my gratitude.

To Janine Jones for the photography that, at key points, assists in demonstrating the thinking offered by this book.

To Steve Cranford and his team at WHISPER globally in New York. A relationship and partnership that began in the most unusual way has become a friendship, and Steve has become the creative genius behind the whole machine. Steve and his team, which includes Tracy Holdeman, are responsible for the new vocabulary, tone, and overall presentation of the book, website, illustrations, and more. I had no way to even begin visualizing what he had accomplished because I didn't know it was possible. (Just before publishing this second edition, Steve unexpectedly had a massive heart attack and died. This book will hopefully be a testament to his memory. I miss my friend along with our conversations and plans.) To Suzanne Hurtig at Suzanne Hurtig Design for the design of the interior of the second edition while maintaining much of flavor of Steve's original first edition design.

To my parents, who formed me into the man I am; to my brothers and sisters, who have been supportive while making sure to keep me humble; and to my in-laws, who have become as much a part of me as my own blood. Thank you. (My father Bill, father-in-law Joe and mother-in-law Irene have all also passed since the first edition. I miss them dearly.)

To my children Christopher (Duke), Sammy and his wife Emma, Ellie, Lauren, Ben, and Maggie, I am proud to be your dad. I hope you get a glimpse of the love your mother and I have for you.

To God, whose grace sustains, enriches, and inspires me. All glory that comes from this book goes to You.

Lastly and most importantly, this book is dedicated to my wife, Susie. Susie has celebrated every milestone and gently questioned every breakthrough. She has freely given of herself to give me time to work on this project to the end. Since the opening of the clinic she has been our unpaid office manager and has been asked to sacrifice her time in so many ways. She is my soul mate in so many ways. She is also my best friend, my favorite travel partner, and my partner in the greatest journey we will ever take—this path through life. My name is on the cover, but this is our book.

{ INTRODUCTION

We've had it wrong.

For decades, the healthcare industry has insisted that while it understands chronic back pain, there is no treatment that reliably achieves long-term relief.[1,2] For years, I was part of the medical profession that believed, practiced, and even preached that understanding.

As a doctor, I marched in lockstep with my colleagues as I explained the lack of treatments offering permanent relief to patients suffering from chronic low back pain. Both my colleagues and I saw no other options beyond repetitive treatments offering varying degrees of short-term relief.

After years of treating patients, focused on my obsession with understanding pain, one night after a long day at my clinic, I was alone in my car driving home, puzzling out yet again what I was not seeing. A whisper in my ear inspired me to challenge my long-held assumptions and those of my colleagues.

From that moment forward, the old way of thinking about the human body—how to work out, move through the day, and fully live life in our own bodies—disappeared. Gone too, was the notion that nothing could reliably relieve chronic back pain. My thinking underwent a dramatic shift. I began to treat back pain as a sports medicine doctor.

This book reveals that shift, a fresh way to treat back pain. This new thinking requires new labels—a new and straightforward vocabulary—as a prompt to truly understand your body, properly care for it, and see it as a beautiful instrument performing the music of your life, enjoyed by you and by others.

My whisper of realization inspires a new understanding of your body as the finely tuned instrument with which you are born and grow into—as not only your body but also your Body Guitar®. As with any musical instrument, when out of tune, the result is often unbearable noise rather than sweet music.

Also introduced is Tune Me®, the new medical orchestration for your Body Guitar®, and the Bracing Muscles™, and String Muscles™ controlling your Body Guitar. Along with Stability Gap™ which is a new understanding of compensation. This all is used to explain the new step forward that this book explains, The Body Guitar Theory®.

A new edition of this book has been coming for the last nine years. Almost from the moment I wrote the book, I have continued to discover more about the back and its treatment. There are a couple exercises in the appendix of this book, but this book is not about exercises. This is a concept book. The concept of back pain is complicated. Deciphering which exercise is for each individual patient might be even harder. You need a therapist to evaluate your body and its compensations to accomplish your tuning. Understanding the concepts is the first important step, and it can be accomplished with a book. Exercises need hands-on instruction.

The Body Guitar Theory is an uprise for you. An uprise in caring for your lumbar spine, your body, and your Body Guitar to achieve your liberation from chronic back pain.

To achieve liberation requires an uprising. Achieve yours.

Because we now have it right.

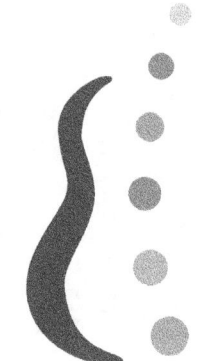

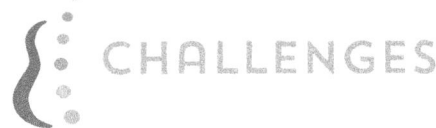 CHALLENGES

Your body is a finely tuned instrument. Like all finely tuned instruments, your body must be properly cared for in order to play the beautiful music it was intended to play. Care for your body and learn to use it correctly, and it will play music that is unique to you—your life song.

—Sean M. Wheeler, MD

As a licensed medical doctor who has practiced medicine for over twenty years, predominantly in the areas of sports medicine and pain management, I have learned a lot about pain and seen firsthand how chronic back pain is treated in this country. Over the course of my career, one thing has become abundantly clear to me about the way the medical establishment treats chronic back pain: it is broken.

The way the medical establishment treats chronic back pain...is completely and utterly broken.

This is no exaggeration, nor do I say this for effect. I mean it literally. The treatment of back pain today is based on flawed premises that all but ensure that many patients receiving treatment for back pain will not see sustained improvement. This is a failure I confront every day in new patients coming into my practice with chronic back pain.

If you have ever had back pain, you know how serious and debilitating this kind of pain can be. You also know how detrimental it can be to your quality of life. Back pain, quite literally, ruins lives.[1,2]

This problem is rampant and growing. Lower-back pain is now the leading cause of disability worldwide. Recent estimates indicate that chronic back pain has resulted in losses totaling more than $100 billion annually.[3,4] Up to 80 percent of Americans will experience significant back pain at some point in their lives,[5,6] and many of them will go on to experience chronic back pain. Annually, 15 percent of all adults are treated for problems related to back pain, such as herniated discs, spinal stenosis, lumbar pain, facet joint pain[7,8]— and the list goes on.

What many, if not most, of these patients have in common is that the medical establishment is failing them. Their doctors are failing them. Our current treatment of back pain is based on misunderstandings and incomplete knowledge. Treated improperly and incompletely, patients with chronic back pain seesaw between treatments and the return of symptoms. When they get pain, they get conservative care. When the pain returns, they get shots. When the pain returns again, they get surgery—only to have the pain return yet again. They are treated but not cured. Sometimes, the treatments ultimately do more harm than good.

As a doctor, seeing my patients not getting any better was hard for me. I knew there had to be a better way. I could see that the system was broken, but I initially didn't understand why. I kept asking myself, "What are we missing here?" As it turns out, the answer was: quite a lot.

I did not start my career in medicine in pain management. My first six years of practicing medicine were spent as a small-town doctor in Kansas. I worked alongside three other doctors from whom I learned the basics of practicing medicine. One of the other physicians, Bob Holt, who was older than me and had a couple more decades of experience, would sometimes stop me when I was making a medical diagnosis or decision about treatment. He would ask me, "Now, what you're doing here? Is this about you, or is this about the patient?"

"Is this about you, or is this about the patient?" What he meant was: Was I making decisions based on patient observations and always acting solely in the patients' interests, or was I making decisions based on assumptions I thought were right and defending those decisions for reasons of ego and pride?

This question was one of his mantras, and it became one of mine. I have since integrated this question into the fabric of my practice of medicine. I think of it as diagnosing my diagnoses, the ultimate exam for my own examinations. I ask the same thing of my fellow physicians, my nurses, and the other medical staff, which probably annoys them to no end, but hopefully it also teaches them what it taught me: how to set your ego aside and focus on the patient.

The other question I like to ask is: "Who is the hero in this story?" This question always focuses me back on the patient. While physicians like to think that we are the hero when it comes to solving a patient's back pain, we are merely an actor in their story. They are the hero of the story, and we need to know our part and remain humble to their pain, their recovery, and their path.

Doctors are, for the most part, bright people. They are highly educated and did well in school. They rely on science, studies, and tests to make diagnoses and are constantly reading peer-reviewed articles and studies to augment their education. The drawback of this is that they become reliant on this pre-existing base of knowledge. Most people have trouble thinking outside of the box, and physicians are no different. But "the box" that physicians find themselves trapped in is one of old thoughts and ideas backed up by new studies that refuse to question established premises. In the medical community, questioning established medical science is akin to questioning the greatness of Walter Payton or Wayne Gretzky—it is heretical. Physicians who would dare to challenge the establishment are rare. Doctors have become personally attached to how they were taught to practice medicine. Thinking outside the box would require doctors to question everything we have been doing for years and admit we were wrong. But we don't want to be wrong. We want to be right.

The problem with wanting to be right is that it can lead to wanting to be right at all costs—even at the expense of the patient. Wanting to be right can slow innovation and allow broken systems and practices to remain in place. As doctors, we should always be questioning how we practice medicine. We should be diagnosing our own profession at all times—after all, if we don't allow ourselves to consider the possibility that something isn't working right, how could we possibly hope to fix or improve it? We have to think outside of the box, and we must go for what some may consider big, new, crazy ideas.

ON BIG, NEW, *CRAZY* IDEAS

In the April 2013 issue of *The Back Letter*,[9] an industry magazine for doctors who work on spinal problems and back pain, there was an editorial note indicating that some in the pain-management community are beginning to question the status quo. The article noted that the Global Burden of Disease Study found that back pain is the single most disabling "disease" worldwide,[10,11] and we are no closer to finding a solution than we were decades ago.[12,13,14] Aage Indahl, MD, a prominent spine researcher, is quoted as saying, "We have been wandering in the wilderness for forty years. We have nothing to show for it."

The article goes on to state that "novel ideas were much more likely to lead to breakthroughs than refining and distilling the research to date," adding that the back pain field has been retreading the same ground over again and getting the same disappointing results. Psychologist Dean Keith Simonton, PhD, pointed out that scientific genius had been responsible for revolutionary leaps forward in many fields. He said that creative researchers often come up with original and useful ideas, but that scientific genius blows the doors off the field. He further said that this is increasingly unlikely in this day and age, suggesting that these scientific leaps are thwarted by the current world of scientific research and that most "cutting-edge" work comes from large, well-funded collaborative teams that already have established research priorities. Dr. Indahl advised, "Let's get crazy. We need crazy ideas." But crazy ideas are not supported in the current environment.

The article closes by offering this solution, a call for more ideas to be put forward in the field: "It makes sense for the spine and back pain fields to...stage events and forums for the expression of novel, off-the-wall ideas—and assess criticism of existing research directions. It would also be sensible for universities, major research institutions, and funding agencies to reexamine the gauntlet of policies that thwart the expression of, and research into, novel ideas and to open the floodgates a little bit."

This closing paragraph struck a chord with me. I created the Tune Me method and wrote this book because the field of pain management is suppressing innovation and creative genius. Though there have been many major advances in the field in the last four or five decades, our current scientific community is set up only for advancement, not major shifts in thinking. We need radical ideas that can solve this crisis because further advancements in doing the same old thing won't get us there. We need a revolution.

To spearhead the revolution, I realized I needed to identify the fallacious premises in the way we have treated back pain in this country and around the world for the last forty years. I had to tackle the flawed ideas we were leaning on so I could get beyond the inertia in treatment that had set in. If I could simply identify those fallacious premises, I could help to offer a solution. To accomplish that, I needed to do two things: diagnose what was wrong with the medical establishment's treatment of back pain and share a new method of rehab with the world by offering a new way for patients to take control of their own pain.

With that in mind, I set about proposing my "crazy idea": the Tune Me method. I have applied this idea in my practice over the years, and it has become a very successful method that I have used to help thousands of patients. I call this method Tune Me because it focuses on bringing all of the parts of the body back into tune with one another. Since your body is a finely tuned instrument, even the smallest problem can lead to a discordant life song. Keeping the body in tune is vital.

Tune Me is a paradigm shift in the treatment of chronic back pain that represents a change in how we view—and treat—chronic back pain. Tune Me leads you out of the box and changes not just your back but also your life.

Tune Me arose from a few simple but troubling questions: Why is back pain so difficult to treat? Why do so many patients not get better or get better only to have their pain return? What are we missing? Why were we treating pain as a symptom while ignoring the underlying causes of that pain? Were we misdiagnosing because we didn't understand the progressive nature of back pain and what causes that progression? How could we diagnose differently and properly? How could we finally understand the progression of back pain and find a solution?

To tackle these questions, I first had to look at myself. When treatments failed, I had to ask myself, What went wrong? Was it because of the patient, the treatment, or the physicians? Finding fault in the treatment would require doctors to rethink the entire way they do business—this is not an attractive option to physicians. The sad and unfair result of this is that, all too often, the patient is blamed. Patients are often dismissed as drug-seeking, attention-seeking, crazy, or simply non-compliant. Anyone seeking treatment for back pain is probably well aware of this sad situation.

But the truth is that the patient is often not at fault—the treatment is, and thus, by proxy, the healthcare providers. If physicians fail to address the fact that our practices are insufficient, then we, too, are at fault. I was tired of being complicit. I was tired of being silent. I knew something was wrong with the way we were treating these patients, and I made it my mission to find the problem.

WHAT LED ME TO DEVELOP TUNE ME

After six years in small-town practice, I was ready for a change. I undertook a sports medicine fellowship, where I was also offered a position in a new fellowship at the hospital in pain management.

To be honest, I wasn't particularly interested in pain management. Who wants to treat people in pain all day? I wanted to focus on treatments and fixing people with sports injuries. But, over time, as I saw how pain negatively impacted people, I became more interested in the management of chronic pain. I realized that "fixing" people in pain actually meant helping them to overcome their pain so that they could get their lives back.

I started out treating back pain like all of the other back pain doctors did. I asked some questions, ordered an MRI, and then gave various symptomatic treatments until one of them relieved the pain.

The more I did this, and the more I learned about the anatomy of the back and the progression of back pain, the more I questioned the way we were treating patients. One of the first things I noticed was that most pain management doctors weren't good at administering physical exams.[15,16]

In my first six years as a small-town doctor, in the only clinic in town, we treated patients with all kinds of ailments. Unless they needed to be sent to a major hospital to see a specialist, we served all of their needs. This experience honed my diagnostic skills and gave me a crash course in providing all kinds of patient care. Our clinic was small, and our lab was limited, so we had to rely primarily on physical exams. This meant getting good at performing a physical exam. These skills are often lacking in modern physicians, who tend to use MRI machines and other tests in lieu of assessing patients by hand. The doctors I worked with were big on putting their hands on patients—and by putting your hands on patients, that's how you diagnose. It is an old-school way of doing things, but it is also effective.

My experience of giving physical exams, coupled with the sports medicine fellowship, put me in a position where I could not only examine my patients' back pain well, but also see the quality of the care that they were receiving—and what I was seeing frustrated me.

Patients weren't getting better, and we, as doctors, were just doing the same old things. I was told to just give patients more injections. This helped for a little while, but the patients would come back when their pain returned worse than before. This wasn't benefitting anyone but me, the physician, and the clinics and hospitals.

In sports medicine, you don't just treat a patient and forget about them. Your ability to get them back to sport is the goal. It becomes a team approach where everyone is pointed in the same direction: return to sport in as good a shape or better shape than they were before the injury. In treating pain patients this way, the bar was raised much higher, and the results were poor. Frustratingly poor.

I knew we needed a new way—a revolution in back pain treatment. I began reviewing all the research on back pain and comparing it to what I was seeing in my patients, and something just didn't add up. All of this research, as well-intentioned as it was, didn't account for the fact that the treatments didn't last. Patients weren't staying better.

Understand that this applies to all treatments. Treatments come and go as we develop new, safer, and better options, but these supposedly better treatments didn't end chronic back pain.

I began reviewing all the research on back pain and comparing it to what I was seeing in my patients, and something just didn't add up.

After forty years of medical breakthroughs in the treatment of back pain, we were simply not treating patients better. As a sports doctor working in pain management, this was untenable to me. The situation had been eating at me for a long time. What were we doing wrong? Again: What were we missing?

MY AHA! MOMENT

One of the more common causes of problems in chronic back pain sufferers is the breakdown of the spinal discs. These discs act as cushions between the vertebrae and are implicated in various kinds of back pain. Throughout all of my medical training, I had been taught that the discs break down due to wear and tear. Of course, this raises the question, why isn't this true for everybody? Some people, regardless of age, have much slower disc break down.

The medical community has decided that disc breakdown is random and predetermined—that some people are simply more susceptible to this wear and tear.[17,18] If this is true, there is little that can be done to prevent the breakdown, and you just treat the symptoms once a problem occurs. This all plays in well with the current approach to managing back pain. After all, as common medical knowledge dictates, the disc just moves and moves until, in some people, it breaks down—and there is nothing you can do about it. The discs have to move, but too much movement can cause them to break down over time.

A year or two after I finished my pain management fellowship and started practicing medicine independently, I was slated to give a lecture to a large group of physical therapists one weekend. In preparation for this lecture, I was poring over some research papers, and I came across an article that caught my eye. It wasn't even the article's main point that caught my attention; it was an aside that piqued my interest. The article discussed how most people develop a lack of blood flow to the lumbar spinal discs by age thirty-five.[19,20,21]

This gave me pause. It stuck with me, and I found myself returning to that article for the rest of the week. I couldn't get it out of my head. It kept me up at night. One thing in particular was bothering me: Why was there no blood flow to the discs? There had to be a reason the disc was set up this way. After all, every part of the human body that is supposed to move gets adequate blood flow.

I was mulling this over in the car on my way home from the office one night. It was about nine o'clock in the evening, and I had had a long day at work and was fatigued. Maybe it was something about being fatigued and having trouble seeing the road—the contrast between the headlights and the darkness was hard on my eyes—that put me in a trance and allowed me to think more clearly, but something clicked for me.

It was suddenly so clear. The discs. The reason they don't get ample blood flow is because they aren't supposed to move. The problem isn't that they move too much in some people—it is that they move at all. The lack of blood flow to the discs indicates that they are supposed to remain stable. That is what separates those whose discs break down and those whose discs don't—the former are unstable, allowing the discs to move. Moving discs also means that the discs are heating up. Anything that moves heats up. The parts of your body that move also have blood flow to take that heat away. If there is no blood flow, you can't take the heat away, and the disc breaks down.

This was an aha moment for me—and it was almost a spiritual moment. Whether you believe in God, evolution, or both, you have to ask yourself—why would the lumbar spine be built this way? Why would God design our backs to break down at this spot over time? How could natural selection not have filtered out a blatant design flaw in such a fundamental part of the body? The answer is that there is no de-

Our backs work perfectly—we are just using them wrong.

sign flaw. Our backs work perfectly—we are just using them wrong.

This moment of recognition started a whole cascade of break-throughs in understanding that revolutionized the way I saw back pain. This fundamental understanding of how discs break down and how the spine must be stable has changed everything about my treatment of the back as a whole. This book is the culmination of all of that change. It all started from that one moment. It set me on the road to discovery. That moment changed the way I viewed chronic back pain and the way I manage it in my patients. I have seen amazing results in my patients as a result of these changes. And it isn't about any one specific treatment—there are many treatments that work—but about making accurate diagnoses and prescribing the correct course of pain intervention and then regaining the stability in the back. The magic isn't in the treatments but in how you approach and use them.

As we move through this book, let us take a brief look at the final result. The end of the book at the beginning, if you will. Your body starts with perfect posture[22]. As we develop, we have a "coming in of the tide" in childhood and adolescence where we are building stability, coordination, and flexibility in waves.[23-27] We all achieve different levels of these goals in this stage, but the goal is thoughtless stability. We have high-tone muscles that stabilize us and allow high-level coordination. We use breath-holding, muscle tightness, and neurological control in thoughtless and seamless integration to augment this stability when needed.[28]

As we age, we have a much slower "low tide" where we begin to lose strength in waves and begin to compensate with the above modalities that are meant to augment our stability but are now asked to provide stability. With back pain, this happens very rapidly. Back pain becomes a disruption of a perfect system of stability that is being used against itself. Back pain sufferers and all of the medical system are fighting a body that is working against itself without them realizing it. This book reveals the problem and a new path to recovery.

My ambition for this book is that it takes my ideas out of the confines of my doctor-patient relationships and brings them to a wider audience and into wider practice. There are millions of people suffering from chronic back pain—and most of them are receiving inadequate care from a broken medical system. I don't want to keep these ideas locked up at my private practice. I want them disseminated far and wide. I want them to change the way doctors work. I want them to benefit patients everywhere.

My other ambition for this book is more personal—it involves you, the reader. I want this book to help you, the individual sufferer of back pain. Whereas changing the medical establishment needs to be a worldwide revolution—there is also a "revolution of one" that needs to occur in each reader of this book. My hope is that everyone who reads this book will begin to fully understand what causes and progresses back pain. While I certainly hope that physicians, physical therapists, and other medical specialists read this book and begin to change the way that we treat back pain in this country, there is no way that you or I can force them to do so. What you can do is take responsibility for your own health by being an informed patient.

You will have to do this anyway. Even with the help of a talented and knowledgeable medical team, patients suffering from chronic back pain will have to remain diligent about keeping their body in tune. This requires making adjustments, both minor and major, throughout the rest of your life. Nobody can do this for you—you have to do it for yourself. No one is saying it is easy, but it is necessary. I want to hear your life song played well, and so do your loved ones. I want to show you the way because no one is going to walk patients down the path to better health. I want to help you take control of your own health. I want to help you sidestep the broken system, which invests in ill-applied treatments that don't treat the underlying problems causing chronic back pain. I want to do all this because, after all, who is this ultimately about? The patient. It's always about the patient. This book is about you. You are the hero in this story.

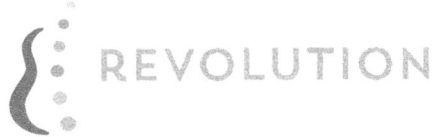 REVOLUTION

The most important kind of freedom is to be what you really are. You trade in your reality for a role. You trade in your sense for an act. You give up your ability to feel, and in exchange, put on a mask. There can't be any large-scale revolution until there's a personal revolution on an individual level. It's got to happen inside first.

—Jim Morrison

What causes a revolution to take hold? Several conditions must be met. First, the situation must be so bad that people rise up and demand change. There also has to be a spark that incites people to take action. Finally, there needs to be a viable alternative to the status quo. People will wallow in the mud all day long and endure all kinds of suffering if no one shows them a better alternative. Provide a better option, and those same people will band together and change the world. Chronic back pain exemplifies this: a dire situation, a simmering spark, and a need for Tune Me.

When it comes to back pain, the world is looking for a change, the medical community is hoping for a change, and patients are praying for a change. As someone who is reading this book, you probably fall into the last category and know exactly what I mean.

I am happy to announce that change is coming. A revolution is coming.

PATIENTS WANT ANSWERS

> Sufferers of chronic back pain are "boomerang" patients—they keep coming back for more treatments.

Patients are frustrated with the lack of effective treatment available to them. I see a lot of patients suffering with chronic back pain. Many of these patients come to me already having received a diagnosis elsewhere. Most have also been treated already, but despite multiple rounds of treatments, they fail to get better.[1] Some of these patients feel better for a little while after receiving treatment, but the pain returns. They come in clutching their MRIs and not understanding why their treatment isn't fixing their problem.[2] They are desperate for an answer to one simple question: Why am I not getting better?

I am not the first doctor to notice that sufferers of chronic back pain are "boomerang" patients—they keep coming back for more treatments. Why, then, is the medical profession not addressing this problem? The answer is that while they recognize the problem, they misunderstand it. Doctors have accepted the premise that this is just the way back pain works. They see back pain as a chronic condition that just naturally returns and worsens, with the only solution being to keep treating it more aggressively.[3]

But it isn't working. What's the answer? A revolution. Patients need a new system.

YOUR DOCTORS ARE JUST AS FRUSTRATED AS YOU

For the most part, doctors are good people who are good at their jobs. They, too, are frustrated with the current state of back pain treatment. They are convinced that if they can just come up with better treatments, they can solve the crisis. Doctors are continually on the lookout for the next great treatment.[4]

Perhaps ironically, we have more and better treatments at our disposal now than ever before. Back pain sufferers try all kinds of treatments and specialists. They see doctors and surgeons, chiropractors, massage therapists, acupuncturists, physical therapists, nutritionists, homeopathic healers, personal trainers, and naturalists. They take herbs, minerals, vitamins, steroid injections, drugs, painkillers, muscle relaxers, and anti-inflammatory medications. They try prolotherapy, traction, manipulation, massages, and rubs. They exercise and go to rehab. They get braces, sleeping devices, and surgeries. They resort to spinal cord stimulators, fusions, stem cells, electrical stimulators, activators, rituals, séances, and more.

The sheer number of available treatment options alone can be dizzying and, ultimately discouraging. Many of the above treatments do work for the management of pain in some patients, but not all patients. For some patients, no treatments work, a fact they don't find out until they have tried them all—no matter how experimental or unproven.[5]

The problem isn't with the treatments themselves. The problem is that treatments are being applied based on misunderstandings and flawed assumptions about how back pain progresses. Doctors don't need new treatments. We need new and better ways of diagnosing patients and utilizing the treatments we already have.

Given how complex back pain and back health are, doctors cannot hope to effectively and efficiently treat patients simply by throwing everything at the wall to see what sticks. The problem with this is that unless a proper diagnosis is made, followed by proper treatments in the proper order, nothing sticks. Physicians and patients need to understand the causes, progression, and intricacies of back pain if they ever hope to find a treatment that works for them.

Again, the answer is a revolution.

RESEARCHERS IN SPINAL CARE ARE FRUSTRATED, TOO

At least once a year, I receive a report that some new research study shows that a well-established treatment for back pain does not produce long-term results. Epidurals that include steroids are no better than ones with lidocaine *after six months*.[6] Epidurals are not effective for spinal stenosis *after six months*.[7] Core strengthening done for six weeks does not produce benefits *at one year*.[8] The list goes on and on. I could probably find a scientific article refuting the benefit of every treatment that has been used in the treatment of back pain.[9,10,11]

What the researchers are proving and re-proving is that something more is wrong than just the pain people are experiencing. Something has changed in the back pain patient that can't be fixed with a procedure or a pill or a surgery or short-term strengthening, or even by getting people back to the regular activities and exercises that they were doing before getting hurt.[12] Something about the post-injury patient has fundamentally changed, and researchers can't put their finger on it. What they are not proving is why chronic back pain exists.[13]

A report from the 2014 National Institute of Health Pain Consortium Research Task Force found that the anatomic basis of chronic back pain is still largely a mystery. The precise anatomic basis for chronic back pain can only be identified in a small percentage of cases, and even in these few cases, there may still be other pain mechanisms and drivers of reoccurring pain.[14]

Research in the field has stalled and needs some "crazy, new ideas" that break from the mold. In short, researchers need a total revolution.

INSURANCE COMPANIES ARE ALSO FEELING THE PRESSURE

Insurance companies are also frustrated with the lack of progress in the medical field. The major insurers are becoming increasingly unwilling to pay for common procedures to treat back pain because these treatments don't produce lasting results. The insurers pay for one treatment after another. This is expensive and ultimately unsustainable.[15]

Imagine if you were an insurance company and had to pay for the care of back pain in your subscribers. You would expect a treatment that worked often, but *nothing has been proven to work*. You would want something that didn't have to be repeated, but *the longer a person has back pain, the more treatments they'll need*.[16] You would want something that was cheap, but *newer, innovative treatments are increasingly expensive and don't appear any better than what we've had before*.[17,18] You would want a final procedure or surgery that you could count on to fix people, no matter the cost, but *surgery, the treatment of last resort, fails just as often as other treatments*.[19,20]

What insurers are paying for is not treatment at all. What they have is a huge group of subscribers on chronic pain meds who also require constant physical therapy or chiropractic treatment and a gamut of procedures, injections, spinal cord stimulators, and surgery. This is driving the cost of insuring these patients through the roof.

Patients with chronic back pain make up the largest population of people on permanent disability. The majority of people who have suffered with chronic back pain for two years or more end up on permanent disability.[21] Insurance companies know this, and they do all they can to avoid having to pay. They know where the longstanding sufferers are headed, and they'll give these subscribers the runaround as long as they can. Insurance companies create rules and regulations about procedures that are exceedingly difficult to meet.[22]

It is easy to vilify the insurance companies here, but the truth is—why wouldn't they want to avoid paying for ineffective treatments that offer little chance of success? Patients and doctors demand these procedures out of desperation, thinking it must be better to try something than nothing.

In the long run, though, this system cannot continue. Insurance companies are increasingly less willing to cover more procedures. Eventually, there will come a point when they won't pay for any of it.

The insurance companies are in need of the same revolution as everyone else.

YOUR PAIN AFFECTS YOUR FAMILY AND FRIENDS, TOO

While I do not want to take the focus off of your pain, I do think it is important to mention how your pain disrupts the lives of those around you. Sufferers of chronic back pain lead a life that is out of tune. Their Body Guitar is playing music that is nothing like what it was destined or designed to play. Other than the sufferer, the people who most often see and feel this imbalance most poignantly are those closest to the sufferer.

It is a testament to the human spirit and human generosity that those around you take as much, if not more, joy in your successes and well-being as you yourself do. When you achieve something great, your loved ones feel joy. The flip side of this is that they hurt when you hurt. The pain that those closest to you feel can rival your own pain, and sometimes even exceed it because they may feel powerless to help you.

Seeing a loved one lose the opportunity for success due to a debilitating chronic illness is difficult to endure. When our friends and family see us hurting, unable to hold down a job, unable to go outside for exercise, sick with side effects from medicines, and unable to improve, they hurt for us. They see us falling into depression and turning into someone whom we weren't before our injury. Our children, grandchildren, spouses, and significant others are perhaps most personally injured by our pain when it prevents us from spending time with them. When sufferers of pain lose their zeal for life, those around them suffer too.

I see my patients with chronic pain leading lives far below their potential, and I think: is this their life song? Not even close. There has never been a more compelling reason for a revolution.

WHY WE AREN'T MAKING ANY PROGRESS

Before a revolution can take hold, there must be a clear alternative option to the status quo. If we are to change course, we must have a reason to expect progress from doing so. This begs the question: Can we do better? Is there a better way to treat back pain? In a word: Yes.

Back pain is certainly difficult to treat, but it is not impossible to treat. Back pain treatments are failing because the problems that patients face are far more complex than what doctors assume.

In short, there are three reasons why we haven't made progress, and they are all related:

1. Back pain leads to instability in the back, which leads to disc and joint breakdown.
2. Back pain is not static—one kind of pain causes another and another. This makes back pain progressive.
3. The muscle weakness that develops following chronic pain is different from what has ever been described before in back pain.

My realization that the discs were not supposed to move changed my entire approach to back pain. I began to see that the initial cause of back pain must be cured rapidly to prevent it from threatening the health of the spinal discs and joints. Pain leads to muscle inhibition, which leads to a change in the balance of muscle stability of the back, which leads to more muscle inhibition. When these muscles are inhibited, the spine is destabilized and leads to disc and joint breakdown, as the spine must be stable.

Doctors are looking for specific and singular causes of pain rather than treating back pain as a systemic problem. Facet joint pain (a term we'll discuss at length later) and disc bulges are not usually isolated events—they are the result or the cause of systemic problems. One kind of chronic back pain leads to other problems because pain actually changes the way our bodies function. You may start out with facet joint pain—as 90 percent of people with chronic back pain do[23]—but, left unchecked, facet pain can progress to disc bulges, discogenic pain (pain from the disc), sacroiliac joint dysfunction, and a whole host of other problems as your pain gets ever worse. When we view back pain problems in isolation, we fail to see how back pain develops and progresses.

Pain further causes muscle weakness that contributes to the cascade of problems that chronic back pain sufferers often face. The problem is that it is a different type of muscle weakness than has ever been recognized by the medical community. It is *Bracing Muscle* weakness.

Bracing Muscles weaken differently, strengthen differently, and function differently than you might expect, as we will see in subsequent chapters. For now, simply understand that, as knowledge of back stabilization requires a revolution in the way we diagnose and treat back pain, acknowledgment of the role of Bracing Muscle weakness in back pain necessitates a revolution in the way we pursue rehabilitation.

If we can address these three issues, it will result in a whole new way of thinking about pain.

Back pain is insidious and progressive. It tends to start as one problem before it leads to another, and then another, and then another—all of this spurred on by muscle weakness. This cycle is hard to break but not impossible. When I developed the Tune Me method, I introduced a Tune Me approach to diagnosis, a Tune Me approach to treatment, and, what will be described in this book, a Tune Me approach to breaking the

Back pain tends to start as one problem before it leads to another, and then another, and then another— all of this spurred on by muscle weakness.

cycle of pain. I am going to show you how to heal your body. But first, I need you to understand the cycle because it is only with this knowledge that you can free your mind and change the way you approach the management of your own pain.

A patient of mine, Sheryl (not her real name), illustrates this point perfectly. Sheryl came to me from a local major medical center because their doctors refused to do more frequent epidurals. Fifteen years previously, Sheryl had been diagnosed with a disc bulge, and she received a series of epidurals with significant improvement lasting for about three months. Then, for the next fifteen years, she received another set of three epidurals every four months. With a history of receiving epidurals on this schedule, Sheryl began to resent that she would feel great for two months, good for one month, and then have to spend one additional month in pain before receiving another epidural. I performed her exam and found no symptoms that fit with a disc bulge diagnosis but instead discovered significant pain over the facet joints in her lower back. When I told Sheryl that a disc bulge was not her problem, I made sure to explain what facet joints were and what pain from facet joints felt like. Sheryl did not want to hear this diagnosis, as she had been having her "disc bulge" treated "successfully" for fifteen years, and she wanted her disc bulge treated.

After listening to Sheryl, instead of continuing the fruitless task of convincing her otherwise, I agreed to administer an epidural with one stipulation: I would administer an epidural only if I could also inject her facet joints. I told Sheryl that she would experience four hours of numbness in her facet joints, and afterward, she would most likely be able to feel whether these facet joints were the cause of her pain. Sheryl readily agreed, convinced that I had little idea of her particular condition—after all, I wasn't the one who had lived with her pain for fifteen years.

After the injections, I found Sheryl weeping in the recovery room. She told me she already knew that I was right, that her facets were the problem because she felt more relief at that moment than she had at any point in the last fifteen years. I told her I was delighted for her, as this was step one, and that when we saw her back in the office for her follow-up, she and I would discuss where we go from here.

Sheryl did not return again for three months. She came in to tell me she had experienced two and a half months of incredible pain relief but now could tell that the pain was returning. I repeated what I had shared previously, that steroid shots don't fix anything, and now Sheryl listened. She smiled (I think she hugged me at one point) and we scheduled her for another procedure, and the result was the same. But instead of waiting three months to return, Sheryl came back one week later just as she said she would, and she readily began physical therapy just as we planned.

Six months later, Sheryl returned with the same pain, just as before. When I asked her what happened with her physical therapy, she said she had tried physical therapy before, and it didn't help. She admitted that she went to the physical therapy I prescribed only because I was so insistent, but when she got there, and the professionals gave her the same exercises as those she had tried years earlier, she decided it wasn't going to work. However, because Sheryl now respected me at some level, she continued with physical therapy for four weeks.

After feeling stronger at the conclusion of those four weeks, Sheryl quit her physical therapy exercises. I asked her, "And yet, somehow, the pain still came back?" But I already knew the answer. I then spent the next twenty minutes retracing the characteristics of Bracing Muscles, explaining how it would require Sheryl to commit to months of concentrated effort to restore her Bracing Muscle strength, how she had to learn how to quit overusing her String Muscles, and how shots do not permanently fix the pain. Sheryl finally told me that she wouldn't agree to retry physical therapy. I then told her that I was unwilling to administer shots to her once again. Sheryl became angry and left, convinced that she would get what she wanted from another doctor somewhere else.

One month later, Sheryl reappeared in my office to say that she would do anything I asked to relieve the pain permanently. This time, I treated her, sent her back to physical therapy, and instructed her to adopt Tune Me in treating her Body Guitar. Two years later, Sheryl appeared in my office looking tan and fit, and she now had her father, who was suffering from back pain, in tow. Sheryl had successfully restored the balance between the String Muscles and the Bracing Muscles to her Body Guitar and was finally liberated from more than fifteen years of pain.

As with the treatments of Sheryl, the solution to the broken system of treating back pain is not better, more expensive treatments. Lack of treatments isn't our problem. The solution is a revolution in how we think about chronic back pain and pain management. We need a revolution in the way both patients and healthcare providers, as well as medical researchers, approach chronic back pain. Patients and doctors need to come together to make this a reality.

What we should be doing is first making diagnoses that determine the exact problem or problems a patient is facing. Then, once we know what the exact problems are, we can create proper treatments to address the pain. Once the pain is treated, we can begin the process of stabilizing the spine that will bring the Body Guitar back into tune.

THE REVOLUTION IS YOU

Do not let yourself become discouraged. The cyclic return of pain can make patients feel powerless. If you have experienced severe back pain, you know what I am talking about. You can feel constantly at war with your own body, with your doctors, with your medications and treatments. Life begins to feel unmanageable and impossible.

I am telling you now: Take heart, it doesn't have to be this way. If you will invest the time in yourself, you and your doctor can be armed with the tools to help you better manage your own chronic back pain and improve your overall health. You have to realize that the steps involve an accurate diagnosis, treatment that creates a pain-free time frame, and then strengthening of the Bracing Muscles unique to stability.

Tune Me isn't a change you will make and forget—it's a change in lifestyle and an ongoing approach to the health of your back and the rest of your body. By first treating the pain and then focusing on strengthening Bracing Muscles and controlling the String Muscles, it is possible to stabilize the back for good in many people. Yes, you will need to remain committed over time to stay in tune, but it is possible for your Body Guitar to stay tuned.

Treating the pain will probably involve treatments that many sufferers of chronic back pain are familiar with. I approve of whatever treatments help to decrease the pain in a patient so that they can begin to do strengthening methods. If a patient needs shots, or an epidural, or even surgery so that they can do strengthening—so be it. We have to reduce the pain.

But we cannot stop there, which happens all too often. The goal of pain reduction should be to make strengthening and rehabilitation of the unique Bracing Muscles possible. Specific treatments come and go. They all have their place. We don't have a shortage of treatments. But what we need is a new treatment plan. If the pain is reduced, but they still can't tolerate strengthening, then we have to look for more treatments to further reduce the pain.

> **The goal of pain reduction should be to make strengthening and rehabilitation of the unique Bracing Muscles possible.**

THERE ARE NO QUICK FIXES

Before you get too excited, understand that there are no easy answers to back pain. For those suffering from chronic back pain, this book will explain how you got into the predicament you are in and what you need to do to get out of it. But there is no silver bullet for back pain, and living Tune Me requires work, dedication, and commitment on the part of the patient. If you have weakness—and you almost certainly do if you have had back pain for any appreciable amount of time—you need to do Bracing Muscle strengthening. This can take some time due to the nature of these unique muscles in the back. No one can do this strengthening for you. And there are no shortcuts.

The Bracing Muscles in our backs are endurance muscles. These are different from some of the Action Muscles that we use to move our bodies. Endurance muscles get weak quickly—sometimes in a matter of weeks. Unfortunately, the process of strengthening them isn't so fast. I tell patients that they can expect it to take at least six months to begin to regain lost strength, sometimes longer. You have to be in it for the long haul.

After we get your Body Guitar in tune, you have to live Tune Me. Our bodies, when they are working at their best, are much like finely tuned instruments. You have to maintain the discipline to keep your body in tune, just as you would with any other fine instrument. Treating the pain and doing strengthening exercises for many months can get us in tune, but staying there means understanding sympathetic control and continuing daily strengthening exercises as necessary. This needs to become the new second-nature understanding of how to manage chronic back pain. Actually, this applies to all people, whether they currently have back pain or not—an understanding of these practices will help people avoid developing back pain in the first place.

Caring for our bodies is a lifelong endeavor. You need to manage your expectations going in and be prepared to put in the work to see results. When someone wants to lose a hundred pounds of weight, they typically understand that this isn't going to happen overnight—or even over a couple of weeks or months. And yet, this is how people think about chronic back pain. They want someone to fix them, and they don't want to put in the work. Now, I can't blame people for thinking this way because doctors treat back pain like they treat a bacterial infection—as if a few shots are going to clear the problem right up. This gives people false hope and sets them up for failure.

Fixing back pain can seem even more glacial than massive weight loss. When you are losing weight, you can jump on the scale and see that you have improved a little. There is no such scale for muscle weakness—it can take six months or more before you even start to see improvement. You have to commit yourself.

Earlier, I talked about a "revolution of one." This is what I mean. You have to take control of your health here—no one can do it for you. Realizing that the back must remain stable necessitates a fundamental shift in the way that we think of the musculoskeletal system and the way we treat back pain. You have to live out that fundamental shift for yourself. The revolution we need places the burden back on all of us to take ownership over our bodies and care for them. We have to keep them stable and healthy. Your medical team can help you get there, but ultimately, only you can care for your own body.

Treating the pain is necessary, but treating the pain won't fix weakness. An MRI is not going to fix you on its own. Your chiropractor, massage therapist, acupuncturist, and even your doctor are not going to be able to fix you. They can treat your pain and guide you to health—but only you can do the strengthening. Only you can commit to keeping the Body Guitar in tune over the long haul.

Don't let that scare you, though—it should be empowering. Let's not wait for the medical establishment to catch up. Let's each and every one of us start the revolution now.

Empowerment is the whole point of Tune Me. The goal here is to form a new understanding of how your body works and to develop a new relationship with your body and health. I am talking about whole-body health here. It's about lifestyle and holistic care—and self-care. As you will see in this book, problems in the back don't exist in isolation. When the back is functioning properly, different parts of the back work together to keep us stable. When something goes wrong in one area, the whole back is affected.

This is also true of the entire body. Tune Me is, therefore, more than a new plan for treating back pain—though it is that. Ultimately, Tune Me is also a revolution in how we think about, care for, and maintain our whole bodies. After finishing this book, I want you to feel and think about your body differently—as an instrument that must be tuned, adjusted, and cared for. I want you to feel like you understand your body better than ever before. I want you to feel like your whole body works together in a way that you can both understand and control. Yes, this book is about chronic back pain—but first and foremost, it is about cultivating a personal relationship with the instrument that is your Body Guitar.

But before we can begin this revolution, we must first free our minds from all the things we thought we knew about back pain.

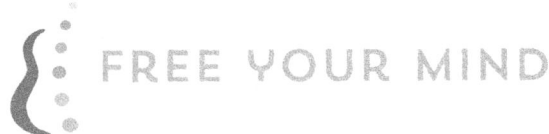

CHAPTER 3

FREE YOUR MIND

As every past generation has had to disenthrall itself from an inheritance of truisms and stereotypes, so in our time we must move on from the reassuring repetition of stale phrases to a new, difficult, but essential confrontation with reality.

For the great enemy of truth is very often not the lie—deliberate, contrived, and dishonest—but the myth—persistent, persuasive, and unrealistic. Too often we hold fast to the clichés of our forebears. We subject all facts to a prefabricated set of interpretations. We enjoy the comfort of opinion without the discomfort of thought. —President John F. Kennedy,
1962 Yale University commencement

What you think you know about back pain is wrong. I am talking to everyone here. This includes patients, doctors, researchers, and insurance companies. Twitter, TikTok, and Instagram influencers and everyone else—all of you. We have held on to myths and clichés for far too long and we must disenthrall ourselves. In this chapter, I hope to help you dispel some serious demons, to free your mind, and to help you unlearn what you think you know about back pain so you can learn anew and the revolution can begin.

FREE YOUR MIND FROM PREVIOUS DIAGNOSES

Patients often come to see me armed with diagnoses they have gotten from other doctors, and they cling to these diagnoses like a lifeline. They tell everyone they meet, "I have this terrible back problem called (insert name here), and that is why I am in the state I am in." They take some joy in having a name for their misery. It is like having a business card that was very difficult to obtain, and they don't want to give it up. They have researched it extensively on the Internet, and because no one has empowered them in any other way, they feel empowered by this knowledge. It belongs to them. It is them. And then I often take it all away. And until they let it go, I have difficulty explaining anything to them. They can't hear a word without running it through the filter of the diagnosis they already have and know so much about. I see their minds working as I try to explain something, and they fit it into their preconceived notions and diagnoses. Don't be this person. Free your mind.

FREE YOUR MIND FROM YOUR MRI FINDINGS

The most common old diagnosis for which new patients come in to see me is some variation of disc bulge/herniation/rupture. These are different terms that the radiologist uses for basically the same thing: the disc is somewhere it is not supposed to be. The specific name doesn't matter. What matters is the effect it is having, or not having, on the nerves in your spine. *(See illustration.)*

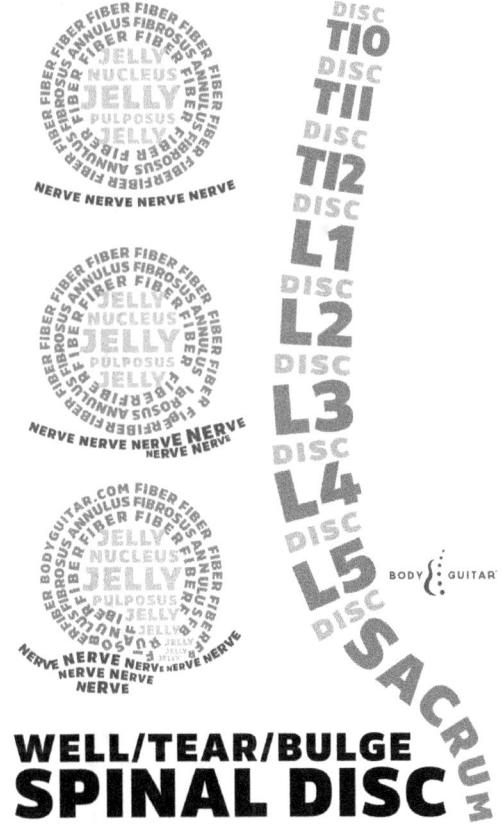

WELL/TEAR/BULGE
SPINAL DISC

One interesting fact about disc bulges is that they are more like-ly to cause pain in the legs than in the back. This is because disc bulges can irritate or damage nerves that go to the legs. So while the discs are in the back, for the most part, they do not cause back pain.[1] Think of it in the same way you would a downed electrical pole in your neighborhood. Your first thought might be whether the power was out in your house—a house that might be a block away from that pole. When you get a disc bulge, it is much the same scenario. It is affecting the nerves that pass by there while going somewhere else. *(See illustration.)*

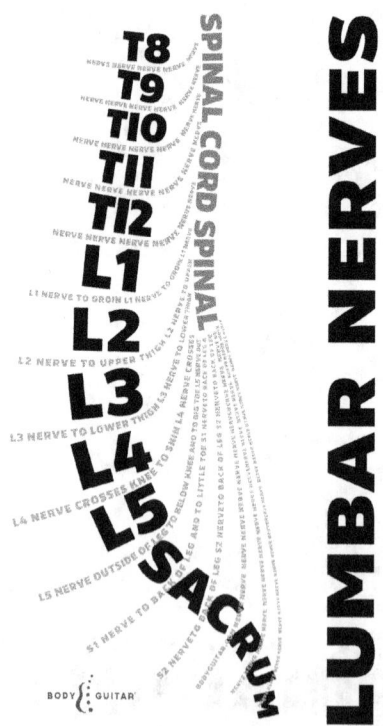

The one exception that I find is a disc bulge at L4/5, which can occasionally cause back pain.[2,3] *(See illustration.)*

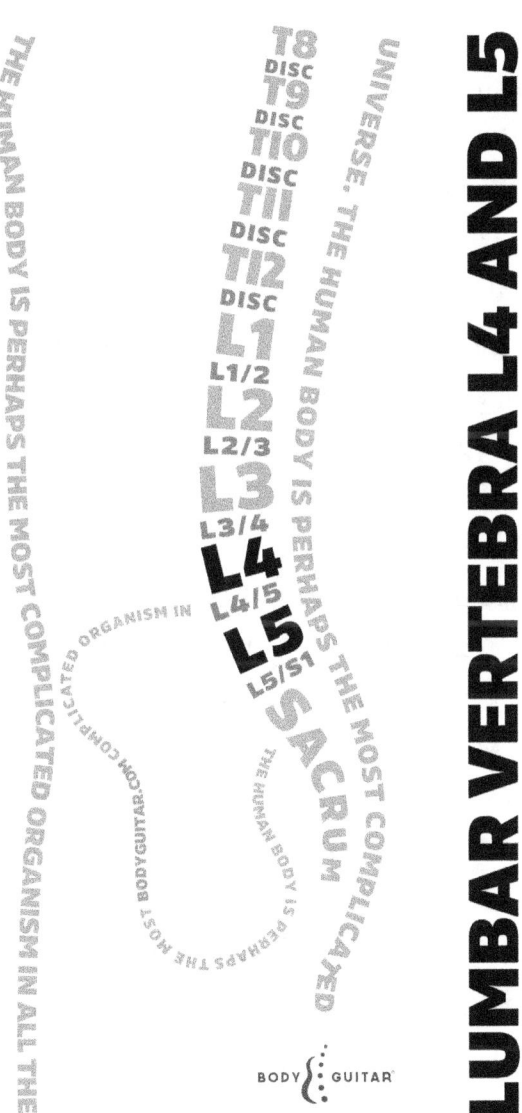

Despite this fact, disc bulges are regularly diagnosed as the cause of back pain. Here's why: Disc bulges are diagnosed by MRI, and MRIs are useful tools. The MRI itself is not the problem. The problem with MRIs arises when they are misused or not interpreted correctly.

MRIs are read and interpreted by the radiologist, who, most likely has never actually seen the patient.[4] The radiologist may only get a one-sentence explanation of the patient's situation if they get any explanation at all. Without proper context, the radiologist doesn't know what to look for. Instead of reporting only relevant information, they report everything they see on the MRI, regardless of its relevance. This creates a poor signal-to-noise ratio that can confuse an accurate diagnosis.

This wouldn't be a problem if the doctor who ordered the MRI had started with a good physical exam, but that isn't what usually happens. Instead, doctors often order an MRI immediately and wait to hear back from the radiologist, who typically does not have any direct contact with the patient and cannot verify that their interpretation of the MRI matches the patient's actual symptoms.[5]

The MRI report is written to look like a diagnosis. However, an MRI is not a diagnosis. It is a tool that requires context and proper interpretation. Many back conditions that show up on an MRI may or may not be the cause of your pain. If the "irregularity" reported on the MRI does not match your symptoms, treating that irregularity will not alleviate your symptoms because the irregularity is not what is causing your pain in the first place.

This is common. Many things considered irregularities on an MRI do not cause pain in most patients. A 2015 study[6] done at the Mayo Clinic found that the prevalence of disc bulging was 30% in participants at age 20, increasing to 84% by age 80. None of the people in this study had back or leg pain.

A 2005 study (Masui)[7] found that there was no correlation between MRI findings of a disc bulge and the continuation of pain in patients. The truth of the matter is that disc bulges, lumbar fractures, spinal stenosis in the elderly, and other MRI "irregularities" are common in people without pain. This is especially true in the case of disc bulges. The MRI can only tell that you have a disc bulge—not if it is the cause of your pain.

The disc is made up of a fibrous shell that surrounds a jelly-like core. When there is a disc bulge, the jelly substance may come out and come into contact with the nerves, irritating them. If it does, the person will experience pain from irritated nerves. If the nerves don't contact the jelly, the patient will feel fine, even if the MRI shows a disc bulge. A disc bulge on your MRI does not mean that the center of the disc is in contact with the nerve.[8]

The noteworthy study was a 1994 study by Maureen Jensen[9] published in the New England Journal of Medicine, where 98 people of all ages without any pain received MRI exams, and 52% had disc bulges. This makes visual confirmation of a disc bulge on an MRI a poor diagnostic tool for pain—and yet MRIs are commonly used to "diagnose" back pain. An MRI can't tell if a disc bulge is causing the pain—only a properly trained diagnostician skilled in giving physical exams and aware of the patient's symptoms and history can do that.

Any of these MRI findings may be the cause of your pain, but they aren't necessarily the cause of pain just because they are present. The findings on an MRI must be matched up with the findings on your physical exam in order to ensure that the patient's symptoms and pain are indeed the result of the finding—and often, they are not.

MRIs are important diagnostic tools. I use them every day for patients with pain. But I do not misuse them. Misdiagnosis can and does occur when an MRI is used in lieu of a good physical exam rather than in conjunction with one. Unfortunately, not all doctors are skilled at giving physical exams or reading MRIs.

Do not let this happen to you. Be your own advocate. Understand the role of the MRI in the diagnostic process, and be sure to ask your doctor if the MRI findings match up with what you and your doctor are observing. In a perfect world, all pain doctors would read and interpret their own MRIs (and not just the report); only use MRIs in conjunction with a fine-tuned exam; and not undervalue the patient's own description of their symptoms. Unfortunately, we do not live in a perfect world. Few pain doctors read their own MRI films, instead relying on the radiologist's report. Few pain doctors are skilled at giving physical exams, which is the direct result of the overreliance on MRIs.

For these reasons, patients must be their own advocates. Make sure that you understand the role of the MRI in the diagnostic process, and be sure to ask the following questions of your doctor before and after your MRI is performed:

- What did you find on my exam that made you want to see an MRI?
- Did the findings on the MRI fit with what you see on my exam?
- Can you explain why you believe these findings are significant when so many people have these findings on an MRI and have no pain?

If your doctor cannot answer these questions to your satisfaction or dismisses you, it may be time to find a new doctor. You want a doctor who will speak up when your MRI results do not match the findings of your physical exam.

Armed with this knowledge, I attack people's misconceptions about MRIs with gusto when the exam just doesn't match what is on their MRI. I explain, I draw charts, I explain again, and before leaving the room, I take all the time necessary to make sure that they understand that the disc bulge, in this case, is not the cause of their pain. Then, my nurse goes in to check them out and returns a few minutes later to inform me that the patient is upset that I am not addressing their disc bulge. Don't be this patient. Free your mind. An MRI is a tool, not a diagnosis.

FREE YOUR MIND FROM THE "TREATMENT ALGORITHM"

I want to take a moment now to consider where back pain diagnoses come from and how they're arrived at. To understand this, you first have to understand a little bit about the general way that the medical community functions, and specifically, how the field of back pain treatment works.

Doctors can be roughly divided into two camps: proceduralists and diagnosticians.[10] Proceduralists, as the name implies, perform procedures. They give injections, perform surgeries, and carry out other procedures. Diagnosticians assess patients to see what is wrong and then give a diagnosis. These two roles do not have to be mutually exclusive, as a healthcare provider can do both, but they describe two separate roles that a physician can fill. Ideally, your doctor will either do both or work within a well-rounded team that is equipped to both diagnose and treat you. Good patient care for back pain starts with a diagnostician making sound diagnoses to which procedures are prescribed.

Unfortunately, this is not the way the medical establishment works with chronic back pain. Rather than diagnosing back pain and applying the right procedure, most back pain doctors instead rely on procedures as a trial-and-error method of diagnosing diseases.[11,12] The majority of doctors working in pain management were trained as proceduralists and not as diagnosticians.[13] Yet we expect providers who specialize in performing treatments to properly diagnose patients by physical exams. For the most part, they can't and so they don't.

They try the first procedure and see if it works—and if it doesn't, they move on to the next procedure until they find something that works. If this sounds wrong, consider that no other field of medicine works this way. That's because there are many problems with this method. It is inefficient; it subjects patients to unnecessary procedures and side effects; and it runs the risk of covering up the patient's pain while the underlying problems continue to fester unnoticed.

You might now be asking yourself: "how did we get here?" The answer is multifaceted and complex, but it can be traced back to historical reasons.

Back pain has been present as long as humans have stood and before. From Herophilus and Erasistratus[14] in the 300s BC to the first sports medicine doctor, Galen, in the 2nd century AD,[15] this pursuit has been an attempt to understand the brain and nerves. From the 1660s with Descartes's *Treatise of Man*[16] to the 1960s and Melzack and Wall's Gate Control Theory of Pain,[17] science has done an extraordinary job of improving our understanding of nerves, receptors, stimuli, the spinal cord, and the brain and how they all play a part in our pain. When pain management became a specialty in the last 50 years,[18] it was in the shadow of these extraordinary scientists and innovators. It was also around the same time that the MRI began to be used in a universal fashion, allowing the spine and brain to be visualized like never before.[19] Naturally, the treatment of pain was directed toward the science of pain. Medications affect receptors and ion channels,[20] injections and surgeries affect stimuli of pain,[21] spinal cord stimulators affect pain nerve impulses,[22] and psychology affects the brain and sensitization.[23] An equally amazing rise of procedures, treatments, and medications has led to medical care that, generations ago, one may have never thought possible.[24] It is a testament to great men and women who have sought to serve humanity by decreasing suffering.

Because the science of pain was one of nerves and disc bulges, pain management became a treatment of nerves and disc bulges:[25] How to identify disc bulges in history, epidurals for disc bulges, and when to send patients to surgery for disc bulges. Spine surgery became the surgical treatment for disc bulges, spinal cord stimulators for nerves, and medications for nerves. Disc bulges and nerves are the basis of all treatments. This fit perfectly with anesthesiologists.

Anesthesiologists are the proceduralists who perform epidurals, along with other highly complex and high-risk procedures used for the care of patients in the operating room. They are among the most specialized doctors in medicine. Decades ago, when epidurals were the primary methods of pain control, anesthesiologists played a major role in pain relief.[26] Patients needed a doctor who could perform epidurals and understood pain medication. Your primary care doctor would make a diagnosis and send you to an anesthesiologist for an epidural. This system worked well for a long time. However, the pain management profession has evolved much in recent years. There are now more procedures and techniques at your doctor's disposal than ever before. Pain physicians now have an expanded repertoire of procedures that they could never have imagined many decades ago.[27-30]

Many patients reasonably assume that the development of more procedures has been coupled with a commensurately more-specialized physical exam in order to ensure that the right procedure is used.

Facets and sacroiliac joints are significant causes of back pain.[31] The problem is that while disc bulges can be treated in a systematic way, facet joint and sacroiliac joint pain are different. They are musculoskeletal problems. To diagnose musculoskeletal problems, one has to develop a musculoskeletal exam. To avoid having to make this dramatic shift, pain management decided to marginalize facet and SI joint pain as an afterthought after disc-related problems were treated or ruled out. The problem is that you can't just throw out every other diagnosis besides disc bulge, because, the MRI is not diagnostic and the pain management treatment for disc bulges is not diagnostic.[32-34]

Back pain is a difficult diagnosis, and there are many components of back pain that look the same. Not only that, but one pain causes another, so the diagnosis becomes as much art as it is science. Back pain diagnosis, along with neck and shoulder diagnosis, is the most difficult musculoskeletal issue any physician may face. After 20 years of treating low backs, my exam and decision-making continue to become more nuanced and complete. This is how it is for all musculoskeletal doctors. Hip, shoulder, ankle, and knee are also all difficult diagnoses.[35-37] The path to becoming a better diagnostician in musculoskeletal medicine is one that leads through asking better questions but must involve improving the physical exam. This is not how pain management chose to proceed. Instead, they convinced themselves that they did not need to do an exam. That the exam was not useful.

You may ask yourself: "How could one entire medical specialty decide that they are the only specialty where the exam is not useful?" The history is complicated, but instead, I will give you the three "studies" that Medicare currently uses to explain why an exam is not done with facet joint pain. The first was a set of questions in 2020 sent to a dozen pain societies and the Veterans Hospitals,[38] which included whether they thought the physical exam was helpful. The second was a 2020 Pain Society consensus statement.[39] A statement which includes this: "The limitations of these guidelines include a paucity of high-quality studies in the majority of aspects of diagnosis and therapy." Therefore, two of the three studies were statements from physicians who don't do back exams on whether the back exam was helpful and included a warning that they didn't really have enough studies yet and that you should take these statements with this grain of salt.

The third was a study that involved 17 studies from 1966 through 2015,[40] where a physical exam was done that showed facet pain, followed by facet injections. After the facet injections, the patient was asked whether they still had back pain without going back and re-examining them. Because there were so many studies, this is not exactly how all of the studies went, but it is how the authors described the results. The authors reported that 25–44% of patients reported that they still hurt. Because so many people hurt afterwards, this suggests that the facet exam was not diagnostic. The fundamental flaw with this study is that patients with facet pain often have pain in multiple areas. In fact, in studies[41,42] of patients after facet joint fusion, where rods and screws are used to hold painful facets together, 35–80% are found to have sacroiliac joint pain. By not going back and reexamining the patient, they have no idea whether the facet joints still hurt, or whether the sacroiliac joint hurts.

These are the three studies used to give pain management permission to take a different approach to physical exams than all of the rest of musculoskeletal medicine. Every other specialty develops a highly specialized exam. Rather than using a more specialized *exam* to diagnose patients, pain doctors have used these type of studies to justify using a highly specialized treatment *algorithm*.

If the MRI shows anything, do a steroid epidural. If there is any pain down the leg, do a steroid epidural. If there is no pain down the leg and no findings on the MRI, treat the facets. If that doesn't work, go back to the steroid epidural, send to a spine surgeon, or place a spinal cord stimulator. If nothing works, treat the SI joint. All along the path, treat with medication. It must be the disc and nerve; it has to be the disc and nerve. If it is anything else, we will treat it, but only after we have treated the disc and nerve. The problems with this treatment algorithm are numerous. This is not good diagnostics. It's not really diagnostics at all. They treat until they (hopefully) find something that works. This delays effective treatment. Worse, the treatment algorithm often results in sometimes major and invasive treatments, such as undergoing surgeries that may be completely unnecessary and may have little chance of helping a specific patient overcome their pain.

The use of algorithms sometimes works in the treatment of other medical problems, such as those in which you are dealing with just one problem. If you have abdominal pain and your physical exam and studies determine that you have an infected appendix, they can stop looking for other causes of your pain.[43] If you have a fever and your doctor finds that you have a raging infection in your bladder, the doctor stops looking for other causes of your fever.[44]

However, the treatment algorithm regularly fails back pain patients because back pain is caused by multiple interlinked problems. First, you have to do a good exam. Then you have to realize that pain in the back starts with one problem and becomes another and another. There is no workable treatment algorithm for that. So how entrenched is the treatment algorithm in the current medical establishment? In a word: very.

I recently had to phone a patient's insurance company. Their physician, who reviews claims had denied approval of my patient's treatment. I had diagnosed pain in both the facet joints and sacroiliac joints based on a physical exam and the patient's symptoms, which were congruent with facet joint and sacroiliac joint pain (both of which will be described soon). So I ordered injections for both areas—the facet joints and the sacroiliac joints. The insurance company denied the claim because standard care—the treatment algorithm—called for doing diagnostic facet injections first and then, if that didn't work, administering the sacroiliac joint injections. I told them that the patient had pain in both of these areas and that I needed to treat both in order to reduce inflammation. I wanted to expedite her transition into physical therapy, which, unlike the injections, would actually cure her pain. I was worried about my patient developing muscle weakness, and I saw no reason not to give both injections simultaneously.

The insurance company physician refused to listen. He maintained that if I numbed both simultaneously, there would be no way to know which had resolved my patient's pain.

"I know what is causing her pain because I did a thorough exam on her," I said. "Her symptoms fit perfectly with both of these diagnoses, not one, not the other, but *both*. We need to treat both together."

"Well, that's not how things are done," he said.

I then explained that she was sent over by a spine surgeon because she had a disc bulge that didn't fit with her symptoms and that if I treated one area at a time, I would never be able to separate these three different diagnoses.

His response was that I should treat the disc bulge first.

"Based on what?" I demanded. "Both the spine surgeon and my

exam suggest that the disc bulge is not the cause."

"Based on the algorithm," he confessed.

What the insurance reviewer did not understand was that treating her facets would barely decrease her pain because sacroiliac joint inflammation is so painful. Conversely, treating her sacroiliac joint would not decrease her pain all that much either because facet joint inflammation is also very painful. Only treating both would result in pain relief. Plus, if I treated one with partial relief that lasted a short time, and then treated the other with partial relief, how would I be able to reliably say that the pain was or was not related to the disc bulge?

This is no anomaly. The system is actually and routinely this rigid and blind to the individual circumstances of each patient. Now, the insurance companies have further mandated that you can only treat two facet levels at a time because they believe that the only way to diagnose facet pain is with diagnostic injections, and if you treat too many at a time, the diagnosis could be confused.[45] They also believe that the facets are the only joint in the body that, if you inject steroids, you have ruined the diagnostic value of the injection.[46] They further believe that you must burn the nerves to the facet joint as the first-line treatment because burning the nerves works for six months to two years.[47] Recent studies have shown that burning of the nerves to the facet joints shut down the multifidus for three years,[48] which (as will be shown later) is a major stabilizer of the spine. Recent findings of multifidus de-innervation call into question the ethics of this nerve burning.

I took a board review course when I was first studying to get board certified as a pain doctor. One of the instructors in the program said that when he saw a patient with back pain, he did three epidurals, and if that didn't work, he did a physical exam. The use of the treatment algorithm and therapeutic procedures to diagnose pain is disturbingly common. This has become the standard care for back pain, and it is an abomination. It is also terrible patient care. I deal with this maddening inflexibility every day as a doctor working in pain management.

You cannot change the medical establishment yourself, but you can free your mind from the shackles of systemic misinformation. There are a number of great pain doctors who are accomplished diagnosticians who don't diagnose and treat pain by the treatment algorithm. You just have to be sure that you have such a doctor. Be sure to ask your doctor what exams indicate that you need a certain procedure. Also, be sure that your doctor is checking that your symptoms match the diagnosis. And whatever you do, don't let yourself become overly attached to an old diagnosis that isn't getting you any better.

FREE YOUR MIND FROM PREVIOUS SUCCESSFUL (OR FAILED) PROCEDURES

Sometimes, patients present from another doctor for a problem they have had in the past. They will quickly inform me what procedure they were given before and request that I perform this procedure. They often don't want to "waste time" being reexamined since they already "know" what is wrong with them. I always deny these requests. I always do a physical exam. I always begin my exam by assuming that the old diagnosis is wrong.

Before you suggest this is hubris on my part, consider that there are a few possibilities that can occur in this type of scenario. First, the diagnosis can be correct, but if so, I will find this on the exam, so no harm, no foul—we can now move forward with treatment and be sure of our diagnosis.

The second thing that can happen in this scenario is that the diagnosis was wrong, but they got a steroid effect that made it look like they were appropriately treated. Steroids have an effect that makes all inflammation feel better. If you get a steroid shot in your foot and your wrist is inflamed, your wrist will feel better.[49] If you get a steroid epidural for a disc bulge, it will have a positive effect on facet joint pain, sacroiliac joint pain, or any other pain because of the steroid.[50] But this does not necessarily mean that you have diagnosed the problem with your back. If you had a good result, it would be temporary either because the disc got irritated again or because you weren't really treating the place that hurt—you just got the collateral benefit. But because you got better, you try another one. When the same thing happens, you try a third. When your pain comes back a third time, you are informed that the epidural proved that your disc was the problem but wasn't effective in decreasing the pain from your disc bulge (which was found on the MRI), and now you need surgery. You have used non-diagnostic imaging (MRI) and partial relief from a non-diagnostic treatment (epidural) and worked your way into a spinal surgery that you may or may not need.

> **This is the human cost of the failed treatment algorithm. Every day, I see people undergoing unnecessary lumbar spine surgery.**

This is the human cost of the failed treatment algorithm. Don't think it cannot happen to you. Every day, I see people undergoing unnecessary lumbar spine surgery.[51] This is why I refuse to use this treatment algorithm, even if you have had some success with a procedure previously, and especially if you are coming to me precisely because your treatment eventually failed.

The flip side of the above scenario is the patient who comes in and refuses a treatment just because they had it before and it didn't work. The problem with this is that they don't consider the fact that several problems or the same problem in several areas may cause back pain. If your treatment failed because you only had one area treated, this isn't exactly a failure of the treatment. Treating one place and still having pain in another is not an adequate trial of the treatment.

Ask yourself: was a thorough exam completed, followed by a thoughtful treatment plan that included *all* of the areas that hurt?

For the majority of patients, this is not how they were prescribed their treatments. For most patients, they arrived at their treatment once they got to its predefined spot in the treatment algorithm that calls for the procedure in question.

The history of sacroiliac joint injections as a treatment for back pain is a prime example of the above problem. As will be discussed later, sacroiliac joint (SI) pain can occur on its own, but in 90 percent of cases, SI pain is the result of pain in another area of the back or body.[52] Back pain causes weakness, which causes a change in the way you walk and move, leading to SI pain. *(See illustration.)*

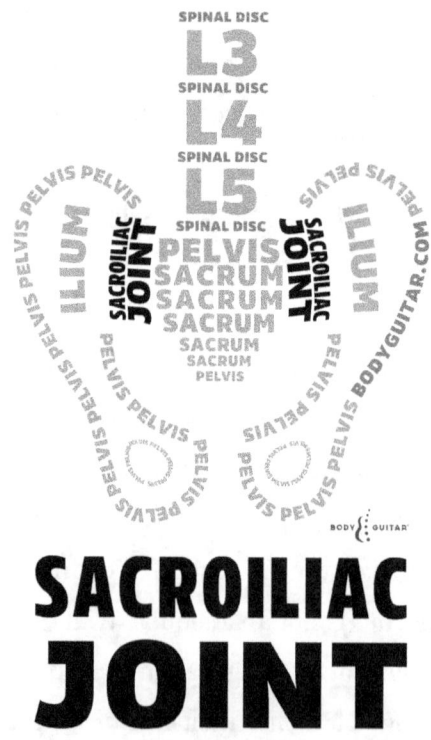

As a patient, it is sometimes difficult to accurately gauge where your pain is coming from. Patients cannot differentiate pain coming from one area or another area a few inches away, especially as it pertains to the buttocks and lower back. So in the 90% of people who have their SI joint treated but have another pain area causing the SI joint to hurt, the back pain continues. This leads doctors to assume that the SI joint was not causing the pain, or otherwise, they think the treatment would have worked. They then move on to the next treatment in the treatment algorithm, even though SI pain was the problem (just not the only problem).

The remaining 10% of people who have sacroiliac joint pain will get better from the treatment, but half of them will have their pain return after three days. Paradoxically, this return of pain occurs because they are getting better. When pain improves, patients begin to walk better. Walking better is important because it requires patients to use the proper muscles for walking. If a patient has been walking in a different way to protect their back for six months or more, returning to walking normally will result in tired and sore buttock muscles.[53] Much like someone who does squats at the gym for the first time in a long time, these patients will experience soreness. This soreness is a necessary hurdle patients must jump in order to get better. It is a long process, but they need to get to where they can walk correctly, using the correct muscles, for the entire day again, which means strengthening the muscles over time. In the meantime, they will experience pain and soreness over the area of the SI joint, which feels much like the pain they had before.

Add all of this together, and we have 90% of patients with SI pain failing treatment because they have pain in more than one place, and another 5% who appear to have failed treatment because walking better causes pain in the area of the SI joint. To a proceduralist, this looks like a 95% failure rate. This high failure rate has led the medical establishment to label most sacroiliac joint treatments as

> **We have 90% of patients with SI pain failing treatment because they have pain in more than one place...**

experimental.[54] These doctors and all of us need to free our minds from failed procedures.

FREE YOUR MIND FROM FUTURE OR BETTER PROCEDURES

Everyone who suffers from back pain hopes for an easy way out. "There has to be some way to make this easier," patients say to me all of the time. Some are even holding out for a better way, a better treatment, a better procedure, a better pill, or surgery that will magically fix them overnight.

Rest assured that there is not going to be some new, better treatment that will make all of your problems disappear. That is certainly not what Tune Me is about. I am not promising you that Tune Me will be easy, so you can dispel the word "easy" from your vocabulary when it comes to recovering from back pain. Tune Me is not easy—but it is effective.

The road to recovery isn't easy because the Bracing Muscles are difficult to strengthen. It takes time and it takes work. New and better treatments will not change this fact, and so there is no reason to wait for them or worry about them. Any new or better treatment would involve decreasing or eliminating pain, but we already have lots of effective treatments for doing that.

The hard part is getting the back stable again. As long as your back is unstable due to Bracing Muscle weakness, your pain is going to eventually return. This is why there are two steps to getting better: treating the pain and getting your Body Guitar back in tune. We may well see better treatments for pain. We are not likely to see better treatments to get you in tune. If we do get newer treatments, they will assuredly take just as much time and dedication as the current therapy because, any way you slice it, retuning your body is about strengthening the Bracing Muscles, and that takes time and effort.

Try learning to play a song on a musical instrument that you have never played. You'll find that it takes time and perseverance, and you will sound terrible for a while. No one can do it for you. But when you get there, you will be very proud of the song you are able to produce.

Relearning to play your Body Guitar is the same way. You will learn to play your life song correctly. But there is no easy way there. You have to put in the work. Free your mind from looking for the easy way out—it doesn't exist.

FREE YOUR MIND FROM FAILED PHYSICAL THERAPY

After diagnosing the patient, I rely heavily on physical therapists. Physical therapy is an important part of retuning the body. The problem that I run into, though, is that not all physical therapists practice in the same way. An excellent inpatient hospital physical therapist will do something completely different from one in an outpatient facility. Different therapists gravitate towards different expertise.

I want to stress that I am not criticizing anyone here. Just because they are not treating back pain in the way that I want does not mean that they are not great physical therapists. It just means that they are not great for this particular problem. My biggest struggle when I see patients from out of town or out of state is to find them effective physical therapy for back pain in their own locality.

When I send patients to a physical therapist, I want them to receive therapy that will strengthen the Bracing Muscles in their back and decrease their sympathetic overload. I have seen some strong patients in my time: bodybuilders, professional athletes, Pilates instructors, laborers, and other people who depend on strength as part of their occupations. These people are not weak as we normally think of that term, but they do have longstanding back pain that has resulted in weakness in particular Bracing Muscles. If these patients do therapy and have the experience that most people get, physical therapy will fail for them.[55-57] This is not because they are not strong enough. It is because they aren't receiving the kind of therapy they need for the kinds of problems they have.

Many of my patients tell me that their past experiences in physical therapy have included treatments such as ice, heat, ultrasound, massage, TENS, traction, and other modalities. They were then given a sheet of exercises to do at home. But when they did these exercises at home, they used their strong muscles and avoided the weak ones, which fatigued their strong muscles and increased their pain. They then went back to therapy and were told to only do the exercises that didn't cause pain, and they slowly decreased to the point of no exercises as all would cause pain. Meanwhile, they continued the modalities at therapy. These helped to decrease the pain caused by the exercises, and by the time they finished with therapy, their pain was almost back to where it was before they started. This is a disaster. The therapist's job is to figure out which muscles are weak and which muscles are strong and being used all day. Why do exercises that strengthen your already strong muscles? These are the muscles you are depending on throughout the day to keep you out of pain. As you fatigue these, your pain will surely increase. But if you strengthen the weak muscles, now you have really done something.

The weak muscles in these very strong patients are the Bracing

Muscles, unique muscles that require a unique approach to strengthening. A physical therapist must find these muscles and show you how to get them to work. Then, they must show you the String Muscles you are compensating with to make up for the weakness in your Bracing Muscles and how to quit compensating. They also must advance you slowly enough that you don't start overusing these String Muscles again.

You can't be expected to do strengthening when you are currently in pain. If someone sends you to physical therapy while you are in severe pain, your therapist can do nothing but modalities.[58] We have to get pain relief to do strengthening. We strive for pain relief, not for pain relief's sake (although it is good) but for strengthening's sake. We need pain relief to

> **Physical therapy trained in Bracing Muscle strengthening is not just important; it is an essential step.**

get strong. If you got pain relief from a treatment and then, when the pain came back, they sent you to physical therapy because another treatment was somehow unacceptable, you have missed your chance. The strengthening needed to be done while you were feeling better. If the pain relief doesn't last long enough to get the strengthening done, you need more procedures done. Everything has to be geared towards giving you enough relief to do the appropriate Bracing Muscle strengthening and decrease sympathetic overload. Then, when we finally get to that much sought-after, elusive, transient pain-free point, exercise sheets without a significant, detailed, hands-on explanation are almost criminal in my mind. Physical therapy trained in Bracing Muscle strengthening is not just important; it is an essential step.

If all these things aren't addressed, you didn't fail physical therapy; physical therapy failed you. Free your mind from the fact that physical therapy will never work. You will never get better without it.

FREE YOUR MIND FROM WHAT YOU THINK IS CORE STRENGTHENING

Everyone is teaching core strengthening these days. In the past decade, we have physical therapists, personal trainers, and others who have all become core strengthening experts. There is an extraordinary number of people who are working on their core and still get back pain.[59,60] The current definition of core muscles has become any muscle from the bottom of your ribs down to your buttocks. So how is this different from Bracing Muscles? Both are high-tone endurance muscles, but Bracing Muscles are static stabilizers (muscles that hold you steady so that motion is able to happen) and core muscles are dynamic stabilizers (muscles that stabilize you during motion).[61] There is a significant difference in these types of stabilizer muscles, and it was necessary to create a new lexicon to describe these differences. By creating the term "Bracing Muscles," I was able to differentiate two mechanisms of stability that needed differentia-tion. Think of it this way: On a tree, the trunk and branches have to have enough stability to stay upright but also enough mobility to move in the wind. These are like core muscles. The roots, however, have to hold the tree in the ground no matter what. These are like the Bracing Muscles. While it is great for roots to have a trunk and branches, the trunk and branches MUST have roots. Core strength can help static stability, but dynamic stability is severely decreased with decreased Bracing Muscle strength.

The Bracing Muscles are muscles that contract before motion. When your brain tells you to tap your foot, the Bracing Muscles will contract milliseconds before any muscle in your leg or foot. When you turn your head or snap your fingers—assuming you don't have back pain—the same Bracing Muscle will contract just prior to the motion.[62] It is not conscious and therefore, it's difficult to control. They are postural muscles that, in the relaxed state, are always work-ing like a spring. Both Bracing Muscles and core muscles are high tone muscles much like springs that stabilize, but Bracing Muscles are inhibited with pain. When you have back pain, the Bracing Muscles quit contracting. When you activate the "fight-or-flight" sympa-thetic system, they are inhibited. Core muscles are not affected in the same way. It is difficult to do core strengthening when you hurt, but it is impossible to do Bracing Muscle strengthening. To get your static stability back, you have to get out of pain, and then build your Bracing Muscle back to the point where it has enough tone to contract all day with your every motion. Then build your core strength to further augment your stability. But building core strength in the face of poor Bracing Muscle strength is a losing proposition. So free your mind from the idea that your core is strong and that it's all the strengthening you need.

FREE YOUR MIND FROM THE NOTION THAT YOU JUST NEED TO GET BACK IN SHAPE

When you have back pain, you lose the ability to exercise in the way you normally would. Many patients tell me that they would get back in shape if they could just get out of pain. I tell them that this is a laudable goal but that they have a lot of work to do before they can even start thinking about getting back into shape. Being in shape is a good thing, but if you are having back pain, being out of shape is the least of your worries.

You have to get the spine stabilized before you can start trying to get into shape. Trying to exercise heavily when your spine is not yet stable is like trying to fly a flag on a flagpole that is poorly set in the ground—it will probably fail. And if it doesn't fail immediately, it will create a ceiling on your exercise such that any exercise past a certain point of fatigue will cause your back to hurt again. People who begin exercising prior to Bracing Muscle strengthening are rarely going to reach their full potential. Your Body Guitar is warped, and we have to get it right before we can play songs. Put the goal of exercising heavily out of your mind for now because you need to focus on your Bracing Muscles first, not your Action Muscles. Free your mind from thinking that you have to get into shape to get out of pain. Your focus needs to be on strengthening the Bracing Muscles first, not general fitness.

FREE YOUR MIND OF THE FEAR OF BACK SURGERY

You are probably reading this book because you never want to have surgery, or if you have had surgery, because you never want to have to do so again. This is a good thought, but it is also narrow-minded.

The treatment algorithm discussed earlier often ultimately leads to surgery. This results in a percentage of people who get exactly the surgery they need at exactly the right time but also a subset of people who end up undergoing unnecessary surgery that provides no real improvement. The number of people who undergo unnecessary surgery is too high.[63] Even one such surgery is too many.

Perhaps you know someone that this has happened to. Surgery on the back is frightening. We have all heard horror stories of people who ended up with more pain and immobility than they had before surgery. A botched surgery can cause permanent damage to your spinal cord, nerves, and body. Add to that uncertainty about whether or not surgery is even needed, and the whole thing can be petrifying.

These are legitimate concerns. However, do realize that surgery is a valid and often necessary treatment. If the right diagnosis is made and other possibilities are first ruled out, then surgery may be appropriate for you. If that is the case, and your rehabilitation following surgery is good, a positive result is likely to occur.

However, surgery is not always appropriate, and it is no magic bullet. It is simply another pain treatment. Even if you have had the correct surgery at the correct time, you can still have problems. Some people do great for a period of time after surgery only to have the pain come back or have pain develop in another area. This pain can be in the same disc, an adjacent one, or anywhere else in the back. When this happens, it does not necessarily mean that the surgery "failed."[64]

Why is this? Because just doing surgery doesn't fix the underlying problem. You have a disc bulge because your back was not designed to move the way it does when the Bracing Muscles are too weak to stabilize the spine. When the muscles are too weak to stabilize the spine, the back begins to move, and this motion causes heat in the discs. This heat causes the discs to break down because they lack adequate blood flow to take the heat away. This process can cause a disc to bulge and irritate or compress the nearby nerve, which is what leads to leg pain.

How does surgery fix the weakness that drives this process? Easy: It doesn't. The surgery fixes the problem that resulted from the Bracing Muscle weakness but does nothing about the weakness itself. So if you do surgery without also treating the weakness, you have a good chance of having the same or another disc heat up and begin to break down again.[65]

Imagine if you have a car that is out of alignment and pulls to the left all of the time. You will have tires that wear out on one side faster than the other side. Your tires will become lopsided, and this will pull your car even further to one side. You may look at your tires one day and notice the uneven wear and think that changing out the tires will stop the car from pulling to the left. If you change the tires without fixing the alignment, the car will now pull to the left less, and you may feel like you made a good decision—until a couple of months later, when the tires start to wear again. Until you get your alignment fixed, your tires will continue to wear out, and you will go poor buying new tires every few months.

This is a lot like the person who gets back surgery but never does any strengthening of the Bracing Muscles. They feel better at first having gotten surgery because they are indeed better, but if they don't fix the underlying cause of the problem they treated with surgery, both problems will reemerge. This is just setting yourself up for another back surgery—or a whole cycle of back surgeries.

Back surgery is serious business, no doubt about it. It is understandable if it scares you. But what you should really be scared of is getting the wrong surgery or doing surgery without the strengthening necessary after the surgery. Appropriate back surgery given at the correct time is a proven treatment. You can free your mind from worrying about back surgery, provided it is done in the right context.

FREE YOUR MIND FROM THE IDEA THAT YOU WILL BE COMPLETELY FREE FROM BACK PAIN

This is one of my least favorite subjects to broach with patients because I do not want to discourage people. Most patients with chronic back pain are driven by the hope of getting rid of it completely. Unfortunately, this is almost impossible. Few patients completely alleviate serious, longstanding back pain.[66]

Please do not let this dishearten you. I think it is important to be realistic, which is why I am upfront with patients so that they do not get discouraged when they don't see the kinds of gains that they want to see. While most people don't completely shed their chronic back pain, they do usually get significantly better. You will probably have to learn to be happy with being significantly better, and that's okay. Any progress is good progress, and significant progress should not be dismissed.

The reason few patients get totally better is because the neural pathways that connect the back and brain become conditioned to the responses they receive. When you develop back pain, every movement requires the brain to figure out which muscles to tighten and which muscles to relax to protect your back from pain.[67]

When this protection mode continues for long enough, it will never completely go away. The brain becomes permanently rewired, and the way you process pain will have changed forever. When you get stressed, your back will hurt. When you get sick, your back will hurt. Pain can manifest in all kinds of ways, and the process is different for everyone. But almost everyone will still experience a certain degree of pain because of this neural rewiring.

Do not think that this means there is no hope. Tune Me may not completely erase your pain, but it can make significant improvements. Tune Me is intended to halt the progression of back pain and decrease your pain significantly so that you can play the life song you were meant to play. Pain relief should still be a goal, but free your mind from the idea that everything is going to be exactly like it was before you had back pain. It probably will not be. But it can be much better than it is now.

● ● ●

There, doesn't that feel better? The mind is uncluttered, unlearned, and unencumbered. We can now build new ideas of what back pain is and how to make the body feel better. But before we can do that, we first need to look at how your Body Guitar got out of tune in the first place.

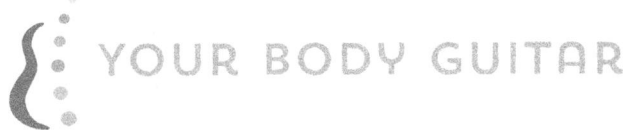 YOUR BODY GUITAR

Body Guitar is a state of mind, a change in attitude, a belief in yourself, and an understanding of your body all wrapped up into one idea.

—Sean M. Wheeler, MD

Have you ever sat near an excellent musician while they were playing and were blown away by what they could do? You feel pulled in, transported to another place by the music they produced, the feeling that they were somehow greater than themselves because of the emotion and feelings they could elicit in the people around them. We all have that power in us. Our inner rock star. It may be how we do our job, or some goal we have set for ourselves, or the way we treat our spouse, significant other, or children and grandchildren, that inspires others to be better than themselves. One person can change the world, but it is so much more difficult when your life is out of tune, and your Body Guitar is not allowing you to play your life song. With back pain, our Body Guitar gets warped and the strings tighten, worsening the situation.

This chapter will first explore how our Body Guitar gets so out of tune before delving into the readjustment process. We will explore how one kind of pain leads to another kind of pain and causes a cascade of problems throughout the whole system of the body. It is this process of pain leading to more kinds of pain that causes the progression of back pain and throws our bodies out of tune.

For this chapter, I have decided to start with facet joint pain and show how this pain progresses. I chose facet joint pain because it is the most common initial site of injury in those with chronic back pain. I could have started on any joint in and around the back or legs and shown how it progresses to other pains, but since the facet joint is the most common starting point, we will begin there. This book is not meant to be a comprehensive medical text, and going through each possible starting point would be burdensome and unnecessary. No matter where your pain began, you will notice similarities between the nature of the progression detailed here and your experience.

Not everyone experiences every step of this pain progression. Even if you are one of the lucky few who only has facet pain or only has facet and sacroiliac joint pain, it is still important to understand the progression because you may later end up further down that path. It is important to understand how the different parts of your Body Guitar are interconnected, which means you still need to understand the whole kinetic chain.

Lastly, please pay attention to the pain story of each affliction, as it is as important as the exam. A back pain diagnosis is difficult enough that I need a history that goes with your pain, an exam that goes with your pain, *and* when I tell you what your day should be like with this pain, you say, "Who told you?" If we go through the first two parts and your pain story doesn't match up, I sometimes rethink the whole diagnosis.

NOT ALL BACK PAIN IS THE SAME

When a patient first comes to a doctor complaining of back pain, all too often, we take a one-size-fits-all approach to treating them, which is the treatment algorithm. Instead, we should approach patients with the goal of discovering the cause of their pain. This cause is often multifaceted and complex.

Most manifestations of lower back pain are attributable to one of five problems:

1. Muscle Strain
2. Facet Joint Pain
3. Sacroiliac Joint Pain
4. Discogenic Pain
5. Disc Bulges

Muscle strain is the most common cause of acute back pain—accounting for over 85% of acute back pain cases.[1] When the muscles of the back are overworked, they go into spasms to protect themselves from further injury.

Facet joint pain, caused by inflammation in the facet joints of the spine, is the second most common cause of back pain. Facet joints connect individual vertebrae, which are the bones that make up the spine. In people with chronic back pain, the facet joints are the site of initial injury in a majority of cases, making it the most common gateway to chronic back pain.[2]

> In people with chronic back pain the facet joints are the site of initial injury in a majority of cases, making it the most common gateway to chronic back pain.

Sacroiliac joint pain (or SI pain, for short) occurs—as the name implies—in the sacroiliac joint. This is where the spinal column connects to the pelvis. This joint is surrounded by ligaments that make the joint essentially immobile—or at least it is supposed to be immobile. When our spine is not properly stabilized due to weak Bracing Muscles, the body compensates by walking differently. Walking in this compensatory way helps stabilize the spine, but it also strains the ligaments around the SI joint until they stretch out and no longer hold the joint steady. The joint was not meant to move, and doing so causes inflammation, which causes pain. SI joint pain can be caused by trauma or genetics, but it is typically the result of muscle weakness caused by another form of chronic back pain. SI joint pain typically represents advanced Bracing Muscle weakness.

A **"disc bulge"** refers to a number of MRI findings in which the soft disc that serves as a cushion between vertebrae bulges out backward toward the spinal canal, often causing pain. A classic disc bulge has many variations, but they generally develop and are treated similarly. Disc bulges are the second most commonly diagnosed cause of chronic back pain, though they are a distant second to facet joint pain. They are also over-diagnosed because disc bulges show up easily on an MRI. Disc bulges cause back pain in about 5% of people,[3] as they mainly cause leg pain, which is significant in itself.

Whereas a disc bulge causes pain in nearby nerves and tissue, **discogenic pain** originates inside the disc itself. Since the pain is coming from the disc, the sufferer hurts anytime they move. Discogenic pain is felt in the center of the back, and it can mimic facet pain, calling for careful diagnosis. Like facet pain and disc bulges, discogenic pain may be triggered by trauma, but the underlying cause is more often destabilization and muscle weakness that leads to the discs heating up. This type of back pain is extremely rare.

These five primary types of pain represent the vast majority of back pain patients suffer. These types of pain are also interrelated and often lead to each other. For the purposes of this book, we are ignoring pain caused by infections of the spine, cancer of the spine, and fractured or broken bones. Those sources of back pain are specific to certain conditions and outside the scope of this book. Instead, we are focusing solely on the main causes of classic low back pain, which are primarily caused by destabilization, heat buildup in the discs, and muscle weakness in the spine.

MUSCLE SPASM

Spasms and pain are the body's warning signals and should not be ignored. Fortunately, back pain from simple muscle strain is mild, responds well to symptomatic treatment, and usually resolves quickly without further problems—typically within a few days to a few weeks.[4] While most muscle strains are resolved easily, muscle strain can be the beginning of a much bigger problem for many people. Continuing to strain your back muscles can injure the joints or discs and lead to chronic back pain. If muscle strain lasts more than a couple of weeks, you must consider whether it is muscle pain you are feeling or the muscle protecting something else that is hurting.

Realize, also, that sometimes this muscle pain is an early sign of Bracing Muscle weakness. I recently have significantly increased my workouts. With that, some weakness in my Bracing Muscle of the right hip has become more evident. This leads to an unconscious compensatory action: breath-holding. This breath-holding leads to String Muscle spasm and, if not addressed, can lead to the whole Body Guitar getting out of tune. All of this will be described later. However, muscle pain is often a sign that we don't have the stability to perform some of the tasks we ask from our bodies.[5]

FACET JOINT PAIN

The facet joints are the site of initial pain for the majority of people with chronic back pain. The facets are joints in the vertebrae that are posterior to the discs and help connect individual vertebral bones, which make up the spine. These joints function like the joints in your knees, elbows, or knuckles, limiting motion with bony surfaces.[6] Unlike the joints in your knees, elbows or knuckles, which provide bony stability, in the neck and back, the bony joints provide little stability, and the muscles are uniquely asked to provide a great majority of the stability. The facet joint's limited range of movement makes them easily injured by moving them farther backwards than their limit or by jamming the joint together.[7] The facet joints' shape and structure prevent them from moving too far. The limited movement prevents your back from twisting too far side-to-side or bending too far backward.[8] When we bend backward, the lower back does little of the motion. The lower back can only bend backward about 10–15% of the way past upright in most adults. The mid-back and neck can bend much farther.[9] Try this out for yourself. Bend backward, slowly and carefully, and notice that most of the flex in your back is in the upper back and neck.

We rarely exceed the range of motion of the facet joints in day-to-day activity, but when we do, the facet joints can be injured in the same way as if you forced a door open too wide, damaging the hinges. This initial damage sets off a biological reaction that causes inflammation in and around the joint. Any joint in your body that gets moved in a direction it wasn't meant to move, or moved beyond its limits, can become irritated, which leads to inflammation.

THE ROLE OF INFLAMMATION IN BACK PAIN PROGRESSION

There are five signs that indicate inflammation: pain, redness, immobility, swelling, and heat (PRISH).[10] If you are experiencing some or all of these symptoms after an injury, it is likely that you are experiencing localized inflammation.

Why does the body do this to itself?

We often think of inflammation as bad, but it is a protective response to injury, harmful stimuli, and irritation. Inflammation is part of the healing process—and without inflammation, wounds and infections would never heal.[11] This is natural and necessary, but inflammation that becomes chronic is a problem because inflammation changes the way we move and position our bodies.[12]

Practicing in a small town in Kansas, I saw many hunters limp into my office complaining of pain in the knee, especially on the second day of September every year. This is because the first day of September is the beginning of dove season. These hunters had spent the previous day hunting in a field with uneven ground. Walking on uneven ground causes the knees to move in unintended and unfamiliar ways, which inflames the knee joint. Usually, the knee recovers in a few hours, but if it gets too inflamed, the whole joint swells up. The treatment here is to prescribe anti-inflammatory medications or a steroid shot and rest the knee until it heals.

The same thing can happen to your back when your spine moves in unintended ways repeatedly. And remember, because the facet joints have limited motion, especially in the lower back, these areas are especially prone to this kind of damage. When the facet joints in the lower back become inflamed, resting the joint until it heals is difficult. Every motion causes the facet joints to move—even just breathing—prolonging the inflammation.

Once the facet joints are inflamed and irritated, a curious thing happens: The muscles in the lumbar spine change to separate the joint's two surfaces, pulling the facet edges apart. The two sides of the joint normally rub against each other, but when the joint is inflamed, movement can further irritate the joint. This process can be set off by any injury—overexertion in the yard, snow shoveling, weightlifting with the back, or any traumatic injuries, such as from a fall or a car accident that forces the facet joints beyond their normal range of motion, injuring and inflaming the area. To protect the facet joints, the brain signals the area to feel pain and the Bracing Muscles are inhibited so they don't hold the edges of the facet together. This process is called arthrogenic muscle inhibition (AMI).[13] We then use the anterior muscles to stabilize the spine, which pulls the spine in a way to hold the facet edges apart. *(See illustration.)*

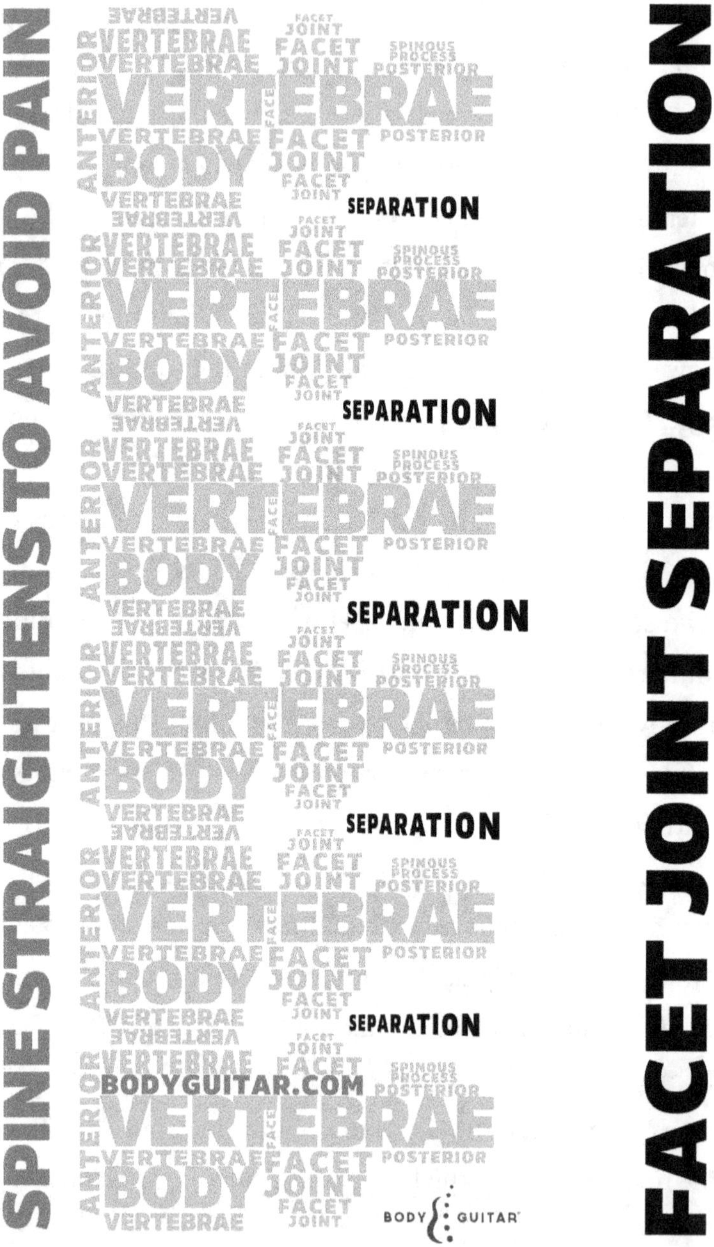
SPINE STRAIGHTENS TO AVOID PAIN
VERTEBRAE
BODY
FACET
JOINT
ANTERIOR
POSTERIOR
SPINOUS PROCESS
SEPARATION
SEPARATION
SEPARATION
SEPARATION
SEPARATION
BODYGUITAR.COM
BODY GUITAR
FACET JOINT SEPARATION

LUMBAR STABILITY

In pulling these edges apart, we are disrupting the delicate balance of lumbar stability. Think of the back like you would an acoustic guitar. If you look through the center hole of the guitar, down inside, you would see wooden wedges and struts that support the shape and stability of the guitar. These are like the Bracing Muscles in our body. In the lumbar spine, these Bracing Muscles are the transverse abdominis on the front of the pelvis and the spinae erector muscles on the back of the pelvis. Both are high-tone muscles that hold the pelvis in neutral, like two ropes on a window washer's platform.[14] The third muscle is the multifidus, a group of muscles that run along the spine and span one vertebrae up to three vertebrae creating small segments of stability. They are high-tone muscles that hold the spine in neutral.[15] These muscles are like springs that allow motion but snap back into place. The two muscles in the back, multifidus and spinae erectors, are stronger than the muscles in the front, transverse abdominus, thereby holding the facet's edges against each other and keeping the pelvis in proper position. Working all together, their thoughtless tone braces the spine for motion; it is the lowest level of stability, as it is postural stability. But by pulling the spine into itself and the pelvis, they are the strongest spine stabilizers and allow the most mobility.[16] We will call these three muscles the Bracing Muscles of the Spine. (See *illustration*.)

BRACING MUSCLES OF SPINE

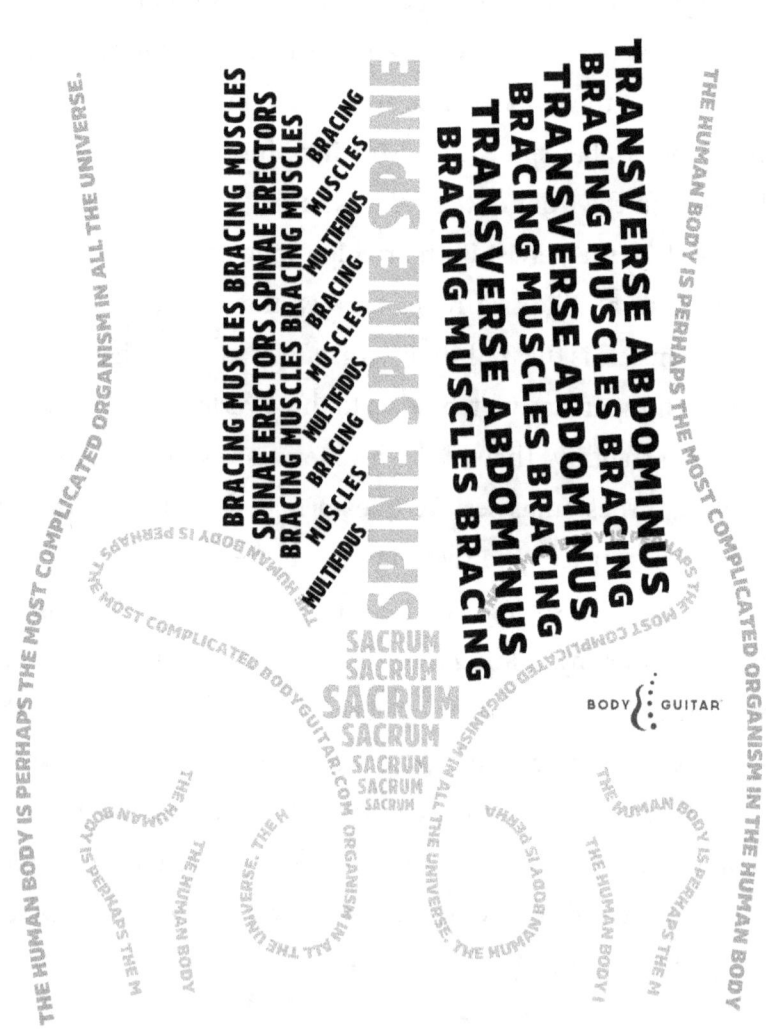

The String Muscles are like guitar strings that run down the fretboard on front of a guitar. These muscles provide balancing stability to the Bracing Muscles, just as a wooden guitar would warp without the strings. Both pull against each other, Bracing Muscles as a spring-like pull and String Muscles as an active muscle pull. Together, this creates a stability in an unstable area of the body. These String Muscles straighten the spine slightly and when fully contracted cause an increased intra-abdominal pressure by abdominal breath holding. The muscles used in this stability are the psoas, iliacus, and quadratus lumborum.[17] The psoas muscle runs from the hip to the diaphragm in front of the vertebrae of the spine. The iliacus runs from the hip to the top of the pelvis behind the psoas, and the quadratus lumborum runs from the top of the pelvis up behind the vertebrae of the spine, to the lowest rib. Essentially, the psoas is in front of the vertebrae, and the iliacus and quadratus lumborum are behind the vertebrae from the hip and pelvis to the diaphragm. *(See illustration.)* From this point on, we will call these three muscles String Muscles of the Lumbar Spine. When we tighten these String Muscles, we create more stability around the spine when needed, but they do so by crossing many vertebrae and pull the vertebrae together, creating large segments of stability. The **unopposed** use of these String Muscles around the spine also causes us to breath-hold. It is not technically "breath-holding' as we continue to chest breathe, but it is restricting our breathing as the diaphragm and pelvic floor are held in position.[18] With the String Muscles, the psoas is a little stronger than the iliacus and quadratus lumborum, which gives our spine a slight forward tilt, pulling the facet edges apart.[19] The hamstring, pulling the pelvis down, also slightly augments this position.[20]

STRING MUSCLES OF SPINE

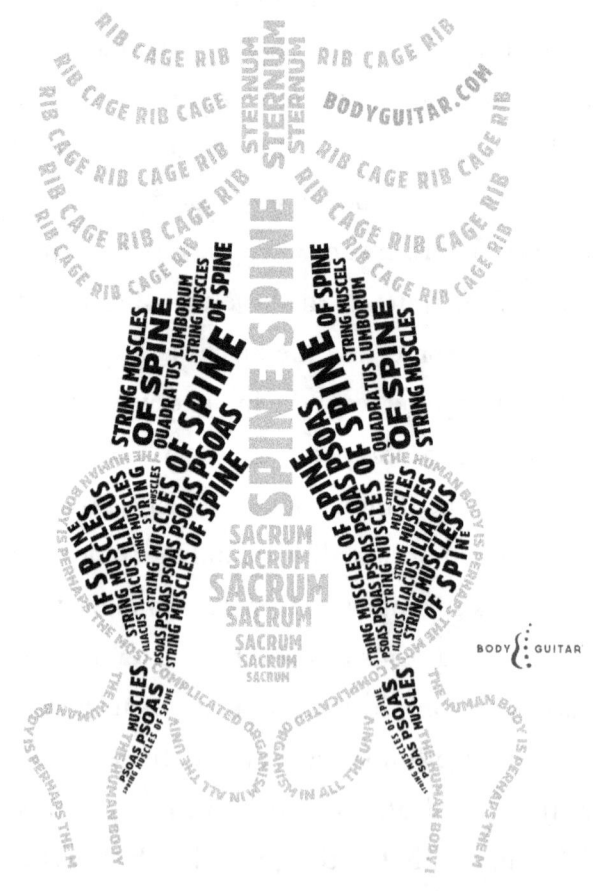

STRING MUSCLES

Many treatments of back pain have been directly related to the treatment of the psoas muscle. Some disciplines of chronic back pain know that the psoas muscle is what they are treating, but many do not. Deep tissue massage will often be targeted to release the psoas spasm.[21] Inversion tables do most of their work by stretching the psoas muscle.[22] McKenzie exercises are both stretching the psoas muscle and strengthening the spinae erectors.[23] Chiropractic manipulation of the lower back causes the psoas muscle to quit spasming.[24] Egoscue Tower is a method to relax the psoas muscle.[25] John Sarno's TMS technique is really a relaxation for the psoas muscles.[26] All provide temporary relief. The treatment of the psoas muscle has been a hinge point for back pain treatment without an understanding of the psoas. So many purposeful and inadvertent treatments of the psoas are well accepted in medicine because of their helpful but rarely curative properties.[27] This is because psoas spasm throws a wrench in a beautifully designed system. As my team began to understand this, what has happened has been a transformation in how we began to rehab low back pain. This started with us asking why the psoas muscle was tight. As we attempted to decipher this problem, it was Shelley Lewis, a talented physical therapist who has helped me throughout my career decipher many problems, who first said, "I think the problem is breath-holding." We then had to try to understand what breath-holding really was and why it affected the psoas muscle. What we found was that breath-holding was a lot like a tight psoas, instead of being the problem, it revealed that the whole system of spine stability was in disarray.

The Bracing Muscles of the spine mentioned above are further inhibited by back pain, as either the facet joints are in pain and need to be separated or we need more space in the spinal canal for disc issues. By straightening the spine, the body attempts to decrease the back pain and switches unconsciously from Bracing Muscles to String Muscles. Because these two muscle groups incrementally inhibit each other, the Bracing Muscles of the spine are inhibited.

The perfectly made system negatively feeds back on itself. The only way to break this cycle is to have a period of time where the back doesn't hurt so that we can quit using the String Muscles. Then, both the pain inhibition of the Bracing Muscles of the spine and the inhibition by String Muscles are removed, and the Bracing Muscles of the spine can start rebuilding tone again.

The problem for many patients is that this inhibition has reached a new level. Bracing Muscles also exist in the hip. The Bracing Muscles of the hip are the gluteus medius and gluteus minimus, which pull the femur up into the joint,[28] and the external rotators of the hip, which pull the femur inward or medially in the joint.[29] These muscles work together to brace the hip for motion. We will now call these three muscles the Bracing Muscles of the Hip. (See illustration.)

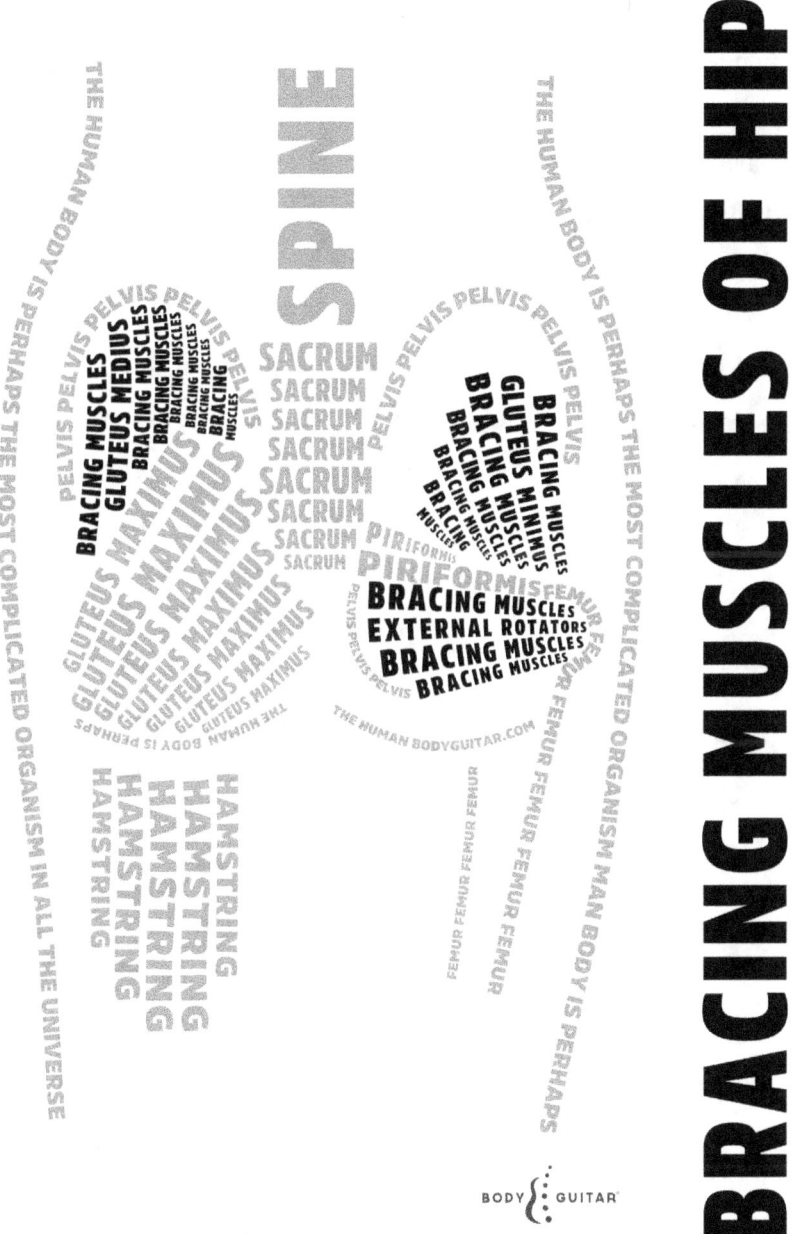

SPINE

SACRUM
SACRUM
SACRUM
SACRUM
SACRUM
SACRUM
SACRUM
SACRUM

PELVIS PELVIS PELVIS PELVIS

PELVIS PELVIS PELVIS PELVIS PELVIS

BRACING MUSCLES
GLUTEUS MEDIUS
BRACING MUSCLES
BRACING MUSCLES
BRACING MUSCLES
BRACING
MUSCLES

BRACING MUSCLES
GLUTEUS MINIMUS
BRACING MUSCLES
BRACING MUSCLES
BRACING
MUSCLES

THE HUMAN BODY IS PERHAPS THE MOST COMPLICATED ORGANISM IN ALL THE UNIVERSE

THE HUMAN BODY IS PERHAPS THE MOST COMPLICATED ORGANISM MAN BODY IS PERHAPS

GLUTEUS MAXIMUS
GLUTEUS MAXIMUS
GLUTEUS MAXIMUS
GLUTEUS MAXIMUS
GLUTEUS MAXIMUS
GLUTEUS MAXIMUS
GLUTEUS MAXIMUS
GLUTEUS MAXIMUS
GLUTEUS MAXIMUS

PIRIFORMIS
PIRIFORMIS

BRACING MUSCLES
EXTERNAL ROTATORS
BRACING MUSCLES
BRACING MUSCLES

PELVIS PELVIS PELVIS

FEMUR FEMUR

THE HUMAN BODYGUITAR.COM

THE HUMAN BODY IS PERHAPS

HAMSTRING
HAMSTRING
HAMSTRING
HAMSTRING
HAMSTRING

FEMUR FEMUR FEMUR FEMUR

FEMUR FEMUR FEMUR FEMUR FEMUR

BRACING MUSCLES OF HIP

BODY GUITAR

With some muscles pulling up and some pulling in, the femur is suspended inside the hip joint by these high-tone muscles, creating less friction with the movement of this weight-bearing joint.[30] When we have back pain, the String Muscles of the lumbar spine pull the femur hard up into the joint and inhibit all these Bracing Muscles of the hip.[12]

When this goes on for months and years, String Muscle dominance leads to atrophy (or shrinking) of these muscles, and even when we are out of pain, activity leads to fatigue of the atrophied Bracing Muscles of the hip. This causes the String Muscles of the lumbar spine to tighten to provide stability to the hip, inhibiting the Bracing Muscles of the spine. And the whole thing becomes a cycle that, instead of seamlessly and thoughtlessly keeping us stable, now seamlessly and thoughtlessly keeps us in pain and unstable. Chronic pain has changed the whole system of stability and used it against itself. Now, instead of using all the forms of stability when needed, we begin to use the String Muscles for everything. *(See Diagram.)*

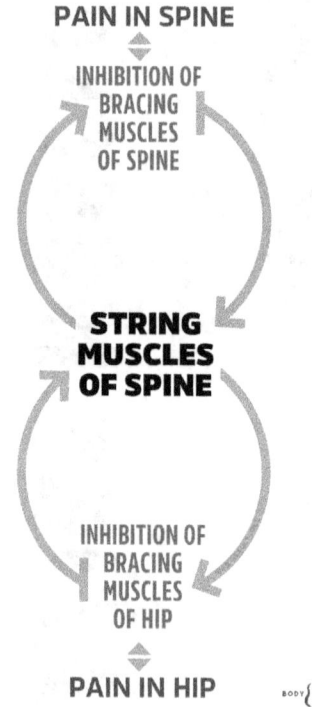

PAIN IN SPINE

INHIBITION OF BRACING MUSCLES OF SPINE

STRING MUSCLES OF SPINE

INHIBITION OF BRACING MUSCLES OF HIP

PAIN IN HIP

When a facet joint injury happens and the String Muscles take over to protect the joint, you feel an initial onset of consistent muscle pain. This initial pain passes over time, but then a particular and predictable pattern of on-again/off-again pain sets in. This cycle is caused by the String Muscles of the back pulling the facet edges apart to decrease the pain, which it does—for a while. However, the muscles must work hard to keep the facets apart to prevent pain, and they are not meant to work this way for extended periods. They are supposed to work in concert with the Bracing Muscles to create stability, and now they are working mostly by themselves. They can do this in a pinch, but they fatigue over time and then spasm, creating a cycle of pain. These are not the spring-like Bracing Muscles that we are talking about. These are Action Muscles, the kind of muscles that move you, that start to spasm in order to protect you.

This constant contraction of the String Muscles shows up as psoas muscle tightness, and all the techniques mentioned earlier relax the psoas. But psoas tightness is not the problem. The problem is that the body is being forced to use the String Muscles for all stability needs of the lumbar spine.

Chronic back pain patients end up with a very common set of findings on exam that reveal this cycle. They will have psoas muscle tightness and quadratus lumborum muscle tightness on exam. Gluteus muscle atrophy and decreased internal rotation of the hip. (This is the motion if you are sitting and want to look at the outside edge of your shoe.) This accumulation of symptoms usually occurs on one side of the body. Often the left side in a right-handed patient, but not always. The gluteus muscle atrophy leads to return of back pain whenever the gluteus muscle fatigues. It eventually leads to breakdown of the balance between Bracing and String Muscle use in the neck, shoulder, calf, and feet. Over time, the sufferer will find that they have issues with the shoulder on the same side as their back pain, knee or hip arthritis on the same side, and even foot pain or Achilles tendinitis on that side, as the pain cycle has led to a cascade of weakness and compensation.

WHEN POOR POSTURE SETS IN

Once the String Muscles fatigue, we have no choice but to adopt awkward postures that keep the facet edges apart while also allowing the muscles to rest. These postures can cause serious problems and lead to more pain. They also look a bit silly. They are:

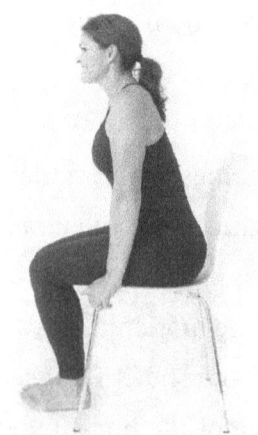

- THE "ARMS HOLDING ME UP" POSE, A SITTING POSE IN WHICH YOU PUT YOUR ARMS OUT TO YOUR SIDES TO SUPPORT YOURSELF IN ORDER TO TAKE PRESSURE OFF OF THE FACETS *(right)*

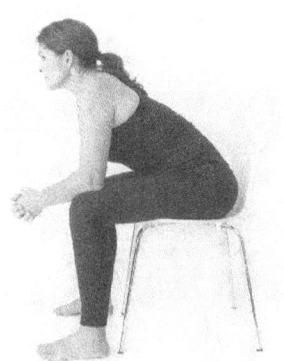

- THE "ELBOWS TO KNEES" POSE,
  ANOTHER SITTING POSE IN WHICH
  ONE BENDS FORWARD AND PLACES
  THEIR ELBOWS ON THEIR KNEES
  (left)

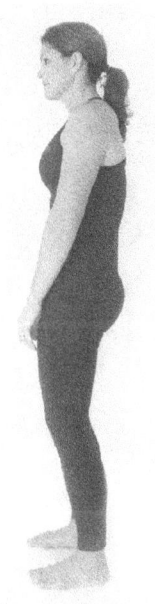

- THE CLASSIC "SLOUCH," IN WHICH
  YOU SINK INTO YOURSELF *(right)*

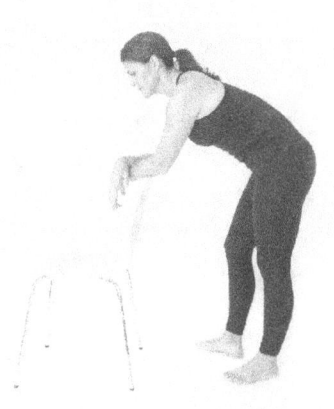

- THE "BENT OVER THE
  SHOPPING CART" POSE,
  SEEN IN EVERY GROCERY
  STORE AND OUTLET STORE
  THROUGHOUT THE WORLD, IN
  WHICH YOU SLUMP FORWARD
  USUALLY LEANING OVER
  SOMETHING *(left)*

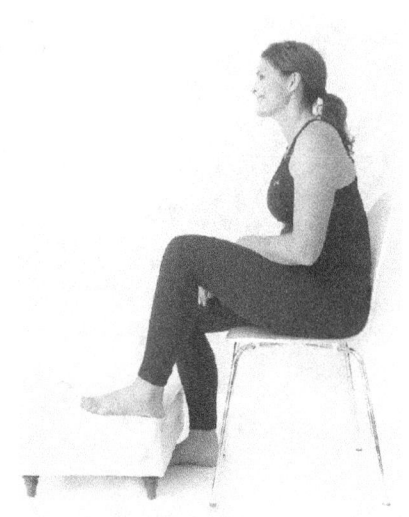

- THE "PUT YOUR FOOT UP ON ANYTHING YOU CAN FIND" POSE, WHICH IS DESIGNED TO CHANGE THE ANGLE OF YOUR PELVIS TO TAKE WEIGHT OFF OF THE FACETS *(right)*

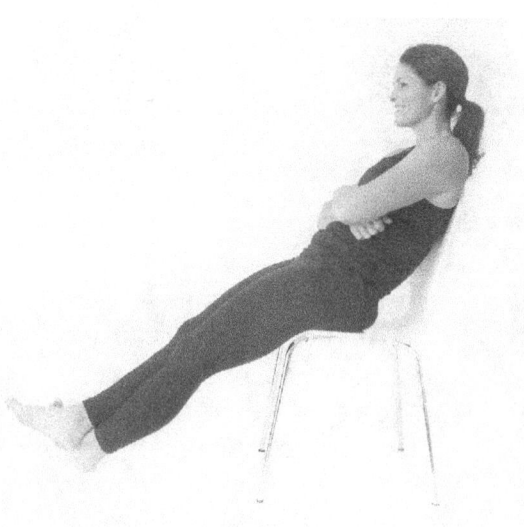

- THE "I'M NOT SLOUCHING" POSE, WHICH IS REALLY JUST SLOUCHING BUT IN A LEANED-BACK POSITION *(left)*

Do you find yourself assuming these poses often due to pain? If so, realize the above poses serve the same purpose: to get the two sides of the painful facet apart once the muscles are too tired to do it on their own. When standing, the spine is stacked and the vertebrae can't be pulled together any more than they already are, so the String Muscles pull the femur into the hip joint and the butt cheeks clamp down. Patients will stand or lie flat and note that it is difficult to relax their butt. When bent over in these positions or in the fetal position, because the Bracing Muscles are inhibited, the String Muscles ratchet down into a shortened position to keep the lumbar spine in a stable position when bent over. Then, when they try to straighten back up, they need to unratchet these muscles back to long again. As there is no Bracing Muscle strength, they are temporarily unstable as they unratchet, so they must bear down to create the necessary stability. If they can't assume these postures for long enough, the String Muscles that hold the facet edges apart become increasingly fatigued until they can no longer do this job, and the joint begins to hurt even more. This is the problem with Action Muscles—they can compensate, but usually not for long.

If you are the kind of person who has to move or walk throughout the day, you are probably going to have to assume more normal positions some of the time. When you do, the muscles must continue pulling the painful surfaces apart. Over time, these muscles, which were not designed to do this all day, become increasingly fatigued and ever more prone to muscle spasms.

This is a progressive process that deteriorates over time. The young and athletic may only have occasional muscle spasms, usually occurring after an extraordinary event, such as after a game, weight-lifting, or other strenuous exertions. Those who are middle-aged or less active may experience muscle spasms only when doing out-of-the-ordinary tasks, such as yard work, snow shoveling, or helping someone move. In the elderly and those with longstanding back pain, even ordinary tasks can cause fatigue in these muscles and lead to muscle spasms. The activities of daily living become a stress on the back muscles, and simply bending forward to turn a doorknob or misjudging the height of a step can cause muscle spasms—and quality of life suffers as a result.

In those with advanced back problems, anything can set off spasms. All too often, it's the little things. These patients can some-times get away with lifting heavy boxes but then hurt themselves bending over to retrieve a dropped pencil. They may do fine carrying the laundry basket, but reaching for the last sock still left in the dryer sends them into all-day pain. For people with facet pain, common everyday tasks and movements can ruin their day.

The same process happens in other joints, such as the knees and elbows, but these joints don't present the same special problems and needs as the facet joints. When we injure our knees, we simply stop moving them until the inflammation subsides and the injury heals. A splint or cast can be used to immobilize the joint if necessary.

But the back is different. You actively move your knees, but your back *gets* moved. The back functions as a stabilizer for the entire body, and therefore, it shifts as we move. Moving your arms or legs, even just shifting your weight, all cause the back to move. To test this, try sitting up straight. Now, try to move just your lower back—not your shoulders, not your pelvis, only your back. Hard to do, isn't it?

You can actively move your arms and legs because the brain can tell an Action Muscle, such as those in your arms and legs, to move—and they do so. However, the Bracing Muscles, like those in the back that stabilize the spine, move automatically in response to conditions to prevent passive motion. The Bracing Muscles and String Muscles work together to hold you steady so that you can move. When the brain tells the legs to walk, the muscles in the back first react by adjusting automatically to stabilize the back and hold you upright. When we move our arms and legs, the Bracing and String Muscles are supposed to react to hold us steady.

This understanding of the body's different muscle sets is not new. Leonardo da Vinci was the first person to suggest that the muscles in the spine perform this stabilizing role.[31] He believed that the body's many moving parts required one stable place to allow us to balance: the lower back. This is a somewhat simplified view, of course, but it illustrates the primary function of the Bracing and String Muscle sets and how they interact.

Modern studies have been designed to explore how the muscle sets interact. A groundbreaking study conducted in Sweden (Cresswell)[32] showed that the Bracing Muscles in the back automatically contract a fraction of a second *before* the Action Muscles in the arms and legs. When your brain tells your limbs to move, the brain first automatically tells the Bracing Muscles to adjust accordingly so that you stay upright.

Much to the scientific community's surprise, Cresswell also found that the Bracing Muscles do not fire at all in people with facet pain. Additionally, the study showed that the Bracing Muscles of the spine will not fire while assuming a posture meant to keep the facets apart (like the postures pictured above). When a person develops facet pain, the Bracing Muscles in the lumbar spine literally quit working.

The Bracing Muscles then begin to atrophy (lose size and strength) as this pain and these postures persist and the String Muscles take over. The String Muscles can cause breath-holding, which also increases the stability around the spine, but this is an ineffective way to stabilize the spine, as one cannot breath-hold all the time. Combined with the String Muscles fatiguing, this on-again/off-again stability leads to increased inflammation in the facets as they are not stable, which causes the body to compensate more, leading to more instability and more inflammation. Over 90% of chronic back pain patients[33,34] end up with atrophy of the multifidus and spinae erector muscles on MRI.

Below is a cross-section of a lumbar spine (bread-slice view). This is someone who works in my office and has a history of intermittent low back pain, but not currently. 1 and 2 are String Muscles and are dark because they are strong and have good blood flow. 3 and 4 are Bracing Muscles of the spine and are supposed to be dark but are inhibited by pain and String Muscles, thus slowly losing blood flow. The ligamentum flavum 5 is a ligament that will thicken to try to stabilize the spine if the Bracing Muscles of the spine are weak.

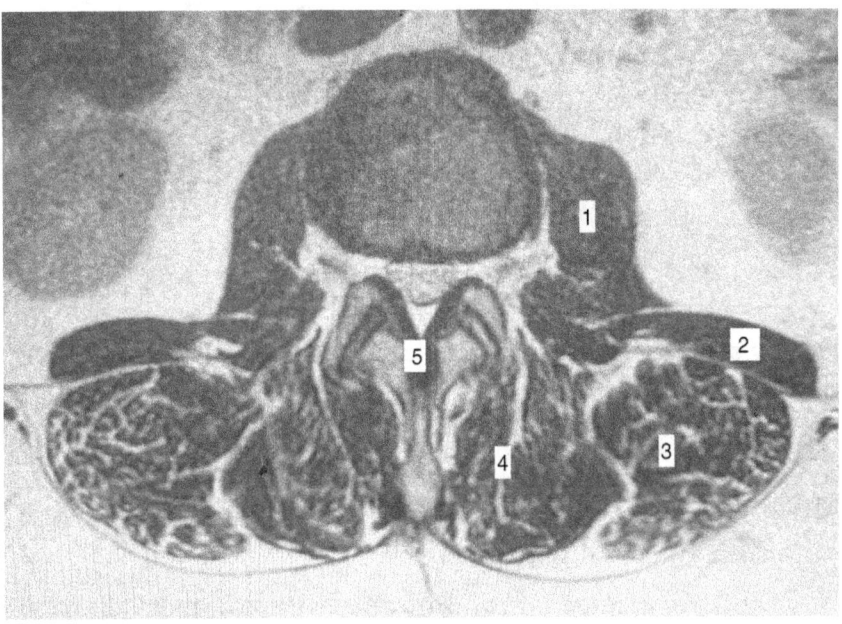

1. PSOAS MUSCLE (STRING MUSCLE)—*strong, dark*

2. QUADRATUS LUMBORUM MUSCLE (STRING MUSCLE)—*strong, dark*

3. SPINAE ERECTOR MUSCLE (BRACING MUSCLE)—*inhibited, light*

4. MULTIFIDUS MUSCLES (BRACING MUSCLE)—*inhibited, light*

5. LIGAMENTUM FLAVUM—*ligament in the spinal canal that thickens when String Muscles take over looks like a V inside spinal canal*

The next two examples are a father and son. The son has great muscle strength, and the father has the most extreme muscle weakness I have ever seen.

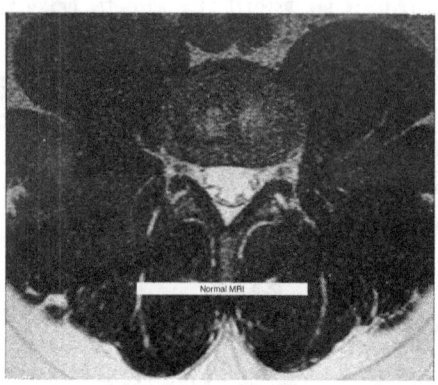 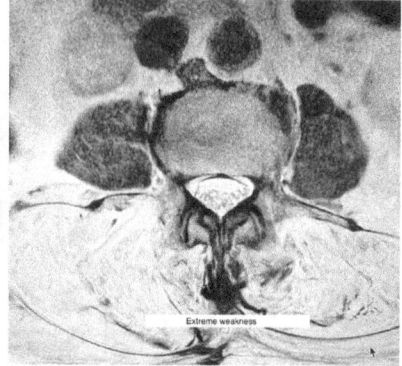

The spring-like Bracing Muscles that effortlessly hold us steady are significantly atrophied. They are the only muscles that can provide stability without overworking, and they are inhibited. All we have left are String Muscles. These muscles cannot work all day and will spasm as they fatigue.

At this point, hopefully, you are amazed at how much one thing causes the other in the lower back and even the body. Just wait; this has only been facets, and we are just getting started.

SACROILIAC JOINT PAIN

For most patients, sacroiliac joint pain, or SI pain for short, is the most advanced form of chronic low back pain. The sacroiliac joint is only a joint in name—it is where the sacrum bone and the iliac bone meet,[35] and it is not meant to move except for nutation, which is what we call the rocking forward and back of the sacrum.[36] Normally, the ligaments and tendons surrounding the SI joint hold it in place, but when these tissues become damaged, the SI joint may become mobile. This usually causes severe pain that can be debilitating and hard to manage[37] *(See illustration).*

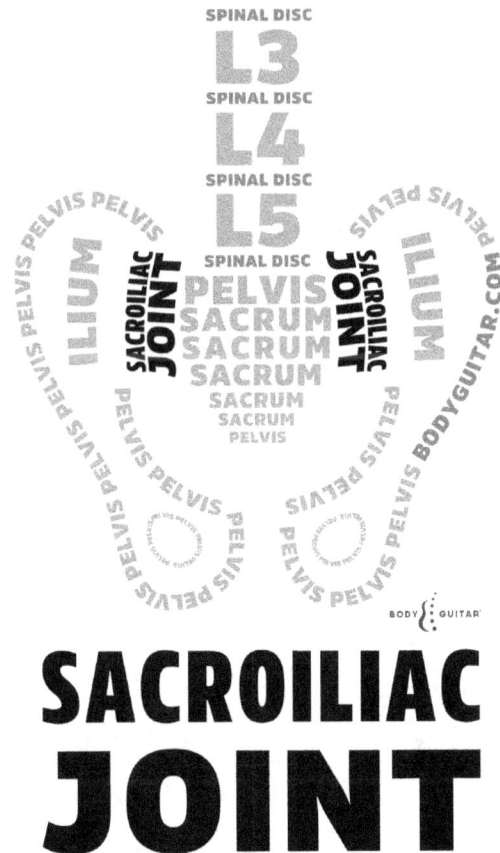

Anything that throws the sacroiliac joint out of alignment can cause pain. In a small number of cases, this develops suddenly from a car accident that smashes the knee into the dashboard, drives the thigh into the pelvis, and knocks the SI joint out of alignment. People with one leg longer than the other sometimes have a limp that puts stress on the SI joint, sometimes leading to pain.[38]

While pain can start in the SI joint, most SI pain is caused by muscle weakness that develops from another form of lower back pain. Anything that stresses the SI joint, if applied long or forcefully enough, can cause the joint to move and become inflamed. SI pain is usually the result of the progression of chronic back pain. Here is how SI pain develops: When you walk, the muscles in your buttocks (gluteus) are supposed to pull your pelvis up to make room for your leg to swing. The pelvis side of the leg that is moving forward rises, and the leg is able to swing freely through the step. When you have facet pain, this rise in the pelvis leads to compression of the facet joint on the same side, leading to increased pain. To prevent this pain, our leg has to swing without the pelvis rising, so we waddle.[39] *(See illustration.)* We sway onto the left leg so that the right hip can rise enough that the leg can swing and vice versa. Most people only begin to do this as they get far enough into their day that the Bracing Muscles of the hip are fatigued, but some do it all day.[40]

This may seem like a good compromise. If it keeps the back stable, who cares if we waddle? The problem is that it places an extraordinary strain across the sacroiliac joint. The constant sway caused by weakness in the Bracing Muscles in the spine and facet joint pain puts pressure on the ligaments around the SI joint with every step taken.[41] Eventually, the ligaments stretch out, which allows the joint to move. The joint isn't meant to move, and doing so causes inflammation and pain.

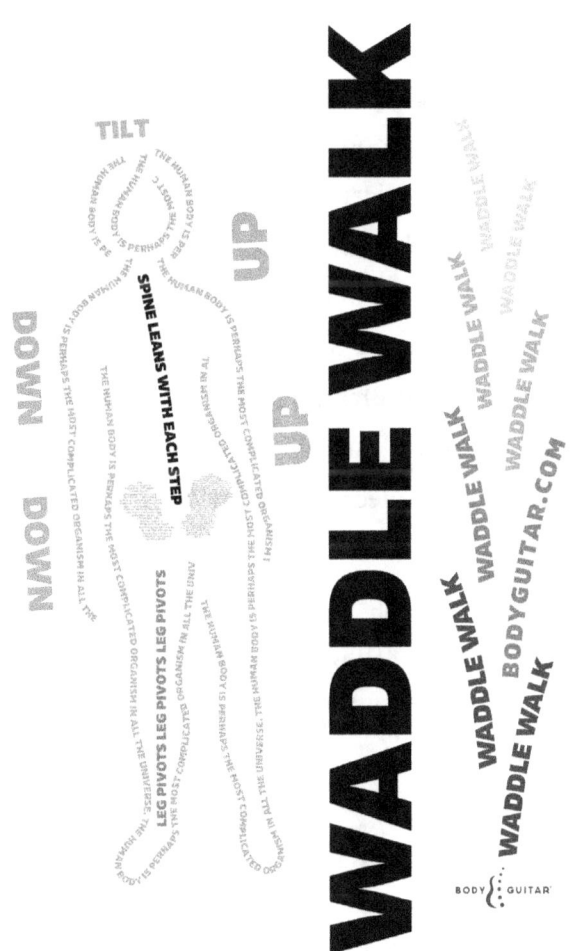

The day that sacroiliac joint pain sets in is significant and typically memorable in the progression of back pain affliction. It is the day when many people shift from being able to modify their activities to prevent back pain to simply experiencing pain every single day, no matter what they do. If you are experiencing SI pain, you are already deep into the progression of chronic back pain and will have to work extra hard to arrest and begin to reverse the situation, though it definitely can be done.

However, it is much more difficult once SI pain sets in, not only because SI pain is an indicator of advanced back pain, but also because SI pain makes it harder to break the cycle of developing pain and weakness. To prevent pain in the SI joint, you have to immobilize it. To immobilize the SI joint, you have to walk with proper form. To do so, you need Bracing Muscle strength sufficient to stabilize the back. To get these muscles stronger, you have to first stop the pain in your facets and decrease String Muscle takeover. Then you have to strengthen the Bracing Muscles of the hips. That's a complex sequence—basically a step-by-step reversal of what got the patient here in the first place. Getting out of pain takes a lot longer than getting into pain. That's because Bracing Muscles weaken quickly, but they re-strengthen slowly.

When people have sacroiliac joint pain, their pain story is specific to them. They have pain if they sit too long. They have pain if they stand too long. They have pain if they walk too long or even lie down too long. Sufferers of SI pain find themselves standing on one leg and then the other. Holding something in one arm hurts. Crossing their legs to tie their shoes sometimes hurts, and sometimes doesn't hurt. If this doesn't sound like you, you probably don't have SI joint pain—at least, not yet.[42] The pain from an SI joint often refers to the back of your knee. This makes it seem like a disc bulge, but no disc bulge refers pain only to the back of the knee.[43] SI pain is associated with other pain as well. The same swaying motion that stresses the SI joint also puts pressure on the hip bursas, which are the fluid-filled sacs that serve as cushions between bones, ligaments, and tendons. This pressure inflames the bursa and leads to hip pain.[44] (The same rationale works for the people who insist that this pain is actually gluteal tendonitis and not hip bursitis.)

Swaying also puts pressure on the connective tissue that attaches the hips to the thighs, which are called the iliotibial band or IT band, resulting in pain down the outside of the thighs. Each of these conditions can cause popping on the outside of the hip.[45] (See illustration next page.)

PIRIFORMIS SYNDROME (OR, I PROMISE YOU IT'S NOT A DISC BULGE)

SI joint pain can also cause piriformis syndrome.[46] This syndrome causes pain that mimics the symptoms of a disc bulge, making it difficult to diagnose.[47] (See illustration.)

ILIOTIBIAL BAND

THE HUMAN BODY IS PERHAPS THE MOST COMPLICATED ORGANISM IN ALL THE

UNIVERSE. THE HUMAN BODY IS BODYGUITAR.COM COMPLICATED ORGANISM

HIP BURSA

HIP BURSA

BODY ⸙ GUITAR

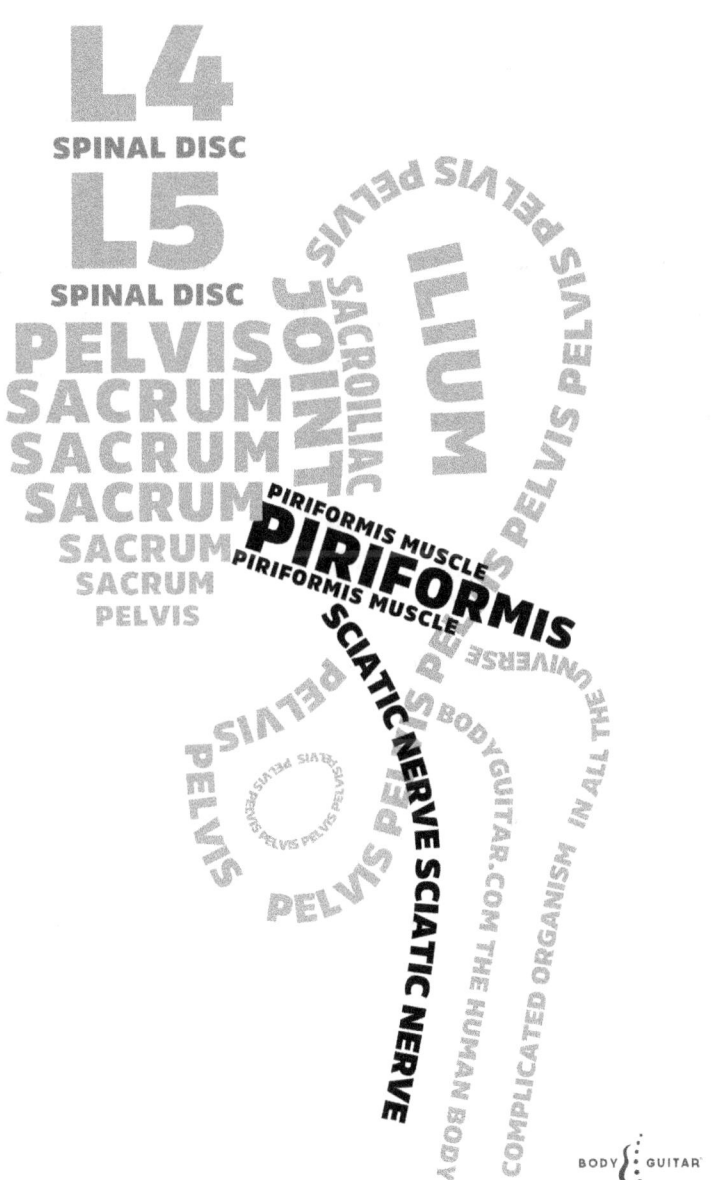

L4
SPINAL DISC

L5
SPINAL DISC

PELVIS
SACRUM
SACRUM
SACRUM
SACRUM
SACRUM
PELVIS

SACROILIAC JOINT

ILIUM

PELVIS PELVIS

PELVIS PELVIS

PIRIFORMIS MUSCLE
PIRIFORMIS
PIRIFORMIS MUSCLE

IN ALL THE UNIVERSE

SCIATIC NERVE SCIATIC NERVE

PELVIS PELVIS

PELVIS PELVIS PELVIS

PELVIS

IS BODYGUITAR.COM THE HUMAN BODY

COMPLICATED ORGANISM

BODY GUITAR

The piriformis muscle runs from the sacrum near the SI joint to the greater trochanter of the hip. There are only four possible reasons why the piriformis muscle is in constant spasm, and the first three are the most common. When either the SI joint or the hip joints are hurting, the piriformis muscle will spasm to protect them.[48] Unfortunately, the sciatic nerve (a major nerve that feeds the legs) runs directly under this muscle. If the muscle irritates this nerve, which it commonly does, you will have pain that mirrors the pain one experiences from a disc bulge. This is a problem because it leads to misdiagnosis of piriformis syndrome as a disc bulge. If you have piriformis syndrome and your MRI shows a disc bulge, your doctors will attribute your piriformis syndrome symptoms to the MRI finding and treat you for the disc bulge. That means a series of epidurals that won't work, followed by a surgery that also won't work because you have the wrong diagnosis.

The third cause is that you can actually have a disc bulge affecting one of the nerves that are included in the sciatic nerve. This is a large nerve comprising the L4, L5, and S1 nerve roots. This nerve is so irritated that any contact from the piriformis muscle hurts and, counterproductively, the piriformis spasms to protect this nerve.[49] Because the disc bulge is easy to find on the MRI, this option makes diagnosis difficult. If we find piriformis spasm and either SI joint or hip joint pain in a patient with a disc bulge, we will often treat the joint pain before the disc bulge as it is a much more diagnostic test.

The last cause, although this diagnosis is often incorrectly made, is that the piriformis will be in spasm because it is trying to do the work of the Bracing Muscles of the hip. The whole pain cascade causes atrophy of the Bracing Muscles of the hip. When they fatigue, the piriformis will try to take over in their weakness and the sciatic nerve is affected. This makes the piriformis much like a String Muscle for the hip.[41]

Piriformis syndrome is just one more example of how one pain leads to another. It illustrates that your body is a finely tuned instrument made up of many mechanical parts that must work in harmony.

DISC BULGES

All movement produces heat. This is easy to observe in the physical world. If you bend a metal coat hanger back and forth repeatedly in an attempt to snap it, the coat hanger gets hot. Rapidly removing a screw from the wall causes it to heat up, and the screw can come out hot enough to burn your fingers. Some of the energy necessary for movement gets converted into heat whenever something moves.[50] The same is true for your body.

Normally, when we move and exercise, the muscles in our back heat up—but when the Bracing Muscles quit firing, the whole area heats up. This includes the bones, ligaments, and most critically, the discs.[51] Our muscles use energy to move, and that motion produces heat. Unfortunately, this heat can be damaging to the discs in the spinal column. Joints, that are supposed to move, have both lubrication to prevent heating and some blood flow to remove accumulated heat.[52] Discs, as they age, have neither.

At the beginning of this book, I described the "aha" moment that led me to the development of the Body Guitar concepts, the Tune Me operating system for our bodies, and the writing of this book. It was the realization that the discs are not supposed to move. I deduced this based on the fact that most adults have no blood flow to the discs. This is evidence that the discs are not supposed to move because movement produces heat, and this heat must be dissipated in order to avoid overheating. The body has many ways of doing this, but the most important one is blood flow.

Anything in the body that is *supposed* to move is filled with blood vessels that both provide energy to the muscles and remove heat from the area.[53] This tells us that if an area of the body does not have blood flow, then that area is not supposed to move. While the discs in the lower back do have small blood vessels feeding them when we are young, these vessels disappear as we age. This partly explains why lower back pain is so heavily correlated with aging. In most people over the age of thirty-five (and almost all smokers), no blood flows through the lumbar discs.[54,55,56] If there is no blood flow, then the heat generated in the discs when the back is not stable cannot be dissipated. And if the heat can't be dissipated, the disc begins to break down.

Recognition of the role heat plays in back pain has informed and transformed the way I treat back pain. And the treatment works. I have seen great results in my patients by addressing the underlying problem of heat accumulation in the discs that develops due to movement.

Picture your spine as a train moving along a set of tracks. In a healthy lower back, the muscles act like tracks, guiding and supporting the train (your spine) as it moves. The discs between your vertebrae are like the connection between the cars of the train, there to provide structure and absorb compressive forces, working smoothly as long as the tracks keep everything in line.

Now imagine what happens when pain or weakness creeps in, and the muscles can't do their job. It's like in the movie The Polar Express when the train comes off the tracks onto the frozen lake. Without tracks (the muscles) to hold it steady, the train (your spine) still has to keep going. But now, the discs are forced to take on way more than they are designed for, not just providing structure and cushioning, but also trying to stabilize the whole system. The discs aren't built for that kind of job, and under this extra strain, they start to break down, leading to pain, injury, or degeneration.

The back is supposed to move when you move. This is why the vertebrae have joints. But the vertebrae and discs are not supposed to move like a coin on top of a dryer—which is basically what happens to your discs when the spinal column is not held steady through passive motion by strong and functional Bracing and String Muscles. Vibrations like these moving through an unstable lumbar spine, especially when left unchecked, are potentially devastating to a back pain patient. If the Bracing Muscles lose function or lack endurance, they cannot keep the discs from heating up. Without strong Bracing Muscles, the back is not stable, and the discs will overheat. This excess heat then causes the discs to break down, causing further pain and destabilization, eventually resulting in debilitation. Thus, what started as muscle strain or facet pain can quickly lead to problems with the discs.

TROUBLE WITH THE DISCS

Between the vertebrae are discs. These are fibrous discs with a jelly-like center that absorb and disperse compressive forces between the vertebrae.[57] These cushions are like the air-filled cushions in the

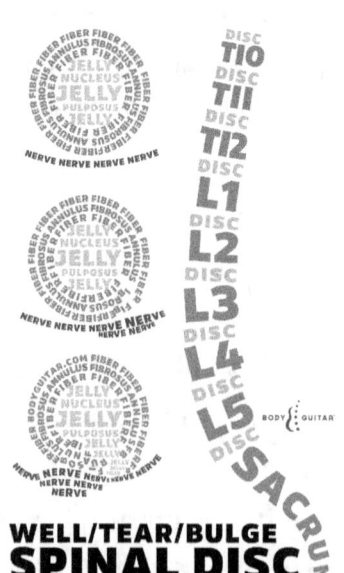

WELL/TEAR/BULGE
SPINAL DISC

heels of some athletic shoes. What they cannot do is withstand the build up of heat. When a disc heats up, it will tear. Micro-tears throughout the disc lead to annular tears, disc bulges, disc herniation, disc extrusion, etc. Disc bulges and disc herniation refer to a number of findings, usually found by an MRI, that show what appears to be an abnormal bulging of the disc—this is due to the leaking of the jelly center out to the edges or outside of the disc itself.[58]

Disc bulges are sometimes the source of back pain. The space that the nerve runs through is called the spinal canal. When a disc bulges the jelly center into the canal, this space is narrowed, and to create more space, the String Muscles will pull the spine straight, inhibiting the Bracing Muscles and creating the cascade of issues much like we saw from facet joint pain. So, while a disc bulge does not usually cause back pain, the change in the way the body stabilizes to protect itself from a painful disc, leads to the same muscle imbalance that occurs from facet pain. This makes disc bugle the second most common cause of chronic low back pain, not because the disc bulge causes back pain, but because of how the spine compensates to protect itself from the irritation of a disc bulge on a nerve. Whether a disc bulge is the cause of your pain is exceedingly difficult to discern from an MRI alone. And yet, all too often, when a patient reports back pain, the very first thing a doctor does is order an MRI before even giving a physical exam. The patient then gets a call back from the doctor's office telling them that a disc bulge of some kind was found and that it is what is causing their pain without the doctor ever checking to see if this is actually the case.

I know this happens because I was guilty of doing this same thing for the first ten years of my medical career. After all, that is what I was trained to do. I didn't question what I was told until I realized that less than half of my patients who showed a disc bulge on the MRI actually had symptoms specific to a disc bulge.

The MRI only tells you that you have a disc bulge—not if it is the cause of your leg pain and definitely not if it is the cause of your back pain. As we discussed in the previous chapter, the majority of disc bulges that show up on an MRI are not associated with any pain, making visual confirmation of a disc bulge on an MRI a poor diagnostic tool for back pain. Disc bulges are common, and they don't always cause pain. But because they are easy to identify, the medical establishment is quick to use them to create a diagnosis without checking to see if the symptoms match up with the diagnosis.

Make no mistake: though over-diagnosed, disc bulges are real. Disc bulges do sometimes correspond with the pain that patients are experiencing, but often, they do not, and an MRI alone is insufficient for telling if a disc bulge is responsible for your pain. You need a doctor who understands the symptoms of a disc bulge and who can verify that the pain you are feeling matches up with the MRI findings.

I have spent the last two chapters mentioning how disc bulges rarely cause back pain but do cause leg pain. This leg pain and dysfunction is important and debilitating. I am not minimizing the nerve pain that is experienced in the patient with a symptomatic disc bulge. I am trying to break down back pain into understandable parts. Doctors call disc bulge-related leg pain radiculopathy, and patients call it sciatica. Radiculopathy specifically means a set of conditions in which one or more nerves are affected and do not work properly.[59] Doctors diagnose radiculopathy by going through the sensation, strength, reflexes, and pain of each individual nerve in the leg and seeing if it is somehow affected. Sciatica means leg pain. It is a symptom rather than a diagnosis. Sciatica is one of the symptoms of radiculopathy but is not the diagnosis.[60] Patients will present and ask me to treat their sciatica and show me their MRI report that shows a disc bulge. I will then go through the exam, looking to see if the nerve pain fits with the disc bulge on their MRI and look for all the other causes of sciatica.

There are many causes of sciatica, and while disc bulge is the most common, a partial list includes: spinal stenosis, spondylolisthesis, peripheral neuropathy, meralgia paresthetica, hip joint pain (both groin and to the knee), SI joint pain, piriformis syndrome, peroneal nerve injury, saphenous nerve pain, facet pain, vascular issues, obturator nerve pain, blood clot, femoral nerve hernia, IT band pain, shingles, pelvis or spine cancer, vertebral fracture, facet cyst, along with Multiple Sclerosis, ALS, and numerous other upper motor neuron and brain diseases.

If that list seems overwhelming, it is because it is meant to be. I want to accomplish two things. First is to let you know that disc bulges and leg pain are a serious pain problem, and my separating back pain from leg pain is meant as clarification and edification only. Secondly, that just because you have pain in the leg and a disc bulge, it does not automatically mean that the two are related. Your doctor needs to be able to differentiate a problematic disc bulge from one that is benign. It is actually the leakage of the jelly-like core that causes the problem. The jelly is great at cushioning the discs, but it is irritating to the nerves. If the disc ruptures and the jelly-like core comes into contact with the nerves of the spinal column, it can produce nerve pain.[61]

However, a disc bulge does not mean that the jelly-like substance will come into contact with the nerves. If a disc bulge is not irritating the nerves, then it isn't the cause of the pain. This means that not all disc bulges cause pain and that an MRI finding of a disc bulge does not automatically mean that it is the cause of a patient's pain.

Currently, the medical establishment treats disc bulges as isolated events—as if they just appear out of nowhere. The truth is that random events can and do trigger a disc bulge, but usually, there are underlying issues that make people susceptible to them. Isolated disc bulges can occur, usually from a car accident, fall, or other severe trauma, but they are far more likely to do so when the back is already out of tune. Often, this is because of untreated pain from the facet joints.

Imagine an old wicker chair that's been left out on your patio for years. Maybe it gave out when Uncle George plopped hard onto it at the family reunion, sending his BBQ plate flying. Was the cause of the chair breaking Uncle George's weight, or was it that you left the chair out in the elements for three years straight? It was both. Uncle George was the triggering event, but the chair's weakness made it possible.

The same is true of your discs. Your disc may have bulged due to a car accident or fall, but you reduce your risk by keeping your body tuned and healthy. In most cases, it is a combination of a trigger and weakness that causes a disc bulge or other back pain. Many of my patients get disc bulges just moving furniture or bending over the wrong way after years of slouching and not exercising. The faulty movement triggered the disc to bulge, but the years of Bracing Muscle atrophy set the table.[62]

DISCOGENIC PAIN

This is also true of discogenic pain, which develops within the discs. Discogenic pain is rarely the initial manifestation of back pain, and it doesn't show up well on an MRI, so it is diagnosed less often than disc bulges, both because it occurs less often and because it is missed more often. In patients with discogenic pain, they will have pain with anything that puts pressure on the disc. Prolonged sitting, especially bouncing in a car can lead to tremendous pain. Walking up or down stairs or hills, or getting up from a chair all puts pressure on the disc. Lying down is one of the only ways to relieve pain.[63] Discogenic pain occurs as a byproduct of the body trying to remove excess heat from a damaged disc by building up blood flow to this disc. Unfortunately, when the body builds small vessels to bring blood flow to the area, it can also build nerves. Your gut doesn't have sensory nerves that tell you how far this morning's meal has passed through you, as your brain doesn't need this information. The same goes for the discs. They can do their job without giving feedback to the brain. But once your body builds blood vessels and nerves to the discs, the brain begins to receive feedback about what is happening there. Any inflammation in the area is translated as pain. Fortunately, I only see discogenic pain due to nerve formation a couple of times per decade.

Both disc bulges and discogenic pain are tricky to treat, especially the latter, and they sometimes require surgery to remove the discs or fuse the vertebrae to get pain under control. As with most problems related to the lower back, prevention is the best treatment for disc bulges and discogenic pain. This means keeping your back in tune and addressing other issues—such as facet joint pain—before they lead to overheating and the breaking down of the discs.

YOUR BODY GUITAR

I have oversimplified the progression of back pain in this chapter. The above description of how facet pain can lead to other kinds of pain is typical of the average chronic back pain sufferer, but there are many permutations and variations of the above. It would be impossible for me to detail them all in the space of this book. However, I don't really need to. The takeaway from this chapter is that lower back pain can manifest as many different kinds of problems, but while these are all distinct problems, they are part of the same progression of chronic back pain. These problems feed off each other and can lead to each other. The end result for too many patients is chronic pain that spreads and gets worse over time. As doctors, we need to stop treating problems in the back as isolated and discrete problems and recognize that one problem leads to another, and another, and another. What I find is that a majority of my new patients have never been given an accurate diagnosis. They have pain, and the only diagnostic thing done was a non-diagnostic MRI. They and their medical team treat the MRI and walk the path of disc and nerve pain, even to the point of life-changing surgery, without ever considering the musculoskeletal causes of pain. When patients don't get an accurate diagnosis and proper treatment that recognizes the progressive nature of chronic back pain, the obvious happens: their pain continues to progress. It worsens and spreads. This, in turn, leads to progressive Bracing Muscle weakness, and String Muscle overcompensation, leading to more problems. This is yet one more vicious cycle that sufferers of chronic low back pain find themselves in. To arrest this crisis, doctors and patients must join together and free themselves from outmoded and broken ways and begin thinking about back pain as interrelated and progressive in nature. It truly is a revolution that has to start with how we think about the progression of back pain.

So, what were my results? We went back to November 2021–February 2022 and looked at every new patient we saw (102 patients) with back pain that we followed over the next 18 months. 36.6% of these patients were 65 years old and above, and 69% were above 50.

Forty-two patients were diagnosed with a lumbar disc bulge requiring an epidural. Seven underwent surgery, and five required a second round of epidurals months after their first successful series. This displays an 83% success rate with an 86% non-repeat rate over the next 18 months.

Twenty patients were diagnosed with lumbar facet pain and were given a steroid injection in their facet joints. One patient needed radiofrequency ablation, and three needed to come back months later for repeat injections. This displays a 95% non-RFA rate with an 84% non-repeat rate over the next 18 months.

Forty patients were diagnosed with both lumbar facet pain and sacroiliac joint pain. Three of these patients were unable to get enough pain relief from injections and required radiofrequency ablation to get through Tune Me. Ten patients needed to come back months later for repeat injections. This displays a 92.5% non-RFA rate with a 73% non-repeat rate.

Zero spinal cord stimulators were placed, and zero patients were given narcotics. One hundred and two patients—seven went to surgery, and four had radiofrequency ablation.

In three patients, we started off treating facets and/or sacroiliac joint and discovered that it was a disc issue, but out of 102 LBP patients, 57 of 60 non-disc related pains were treated correctly from the start. How many would have been incorrectly sent for spine surgery if they started with an epidural? Epidurals in a patient with facet and/or sacroiliac joint pain cause improvement but not cure. Many go on to surgery as they believe it is a disc problem because of the partial improvement. Patients who are given facet and/or sacroiliac joint treatment in a situation with atypical disc bulge symptoms have no immediate improvement and can be rapidly switched to the proper path.

Using steroids in a facet and/or sacroiliac joint led to significant improvement without loss of diagnostic efficacy and allowed us to get through the necessary rehab to create a long-term result. The reason for the increased repeats in patients with both facet and sacroiliac joint problems is that we needed to get stability in their spine and improve pelvis motion with walking. This increased physical therapy requirement led to some patients having a return of their pain before rehab could be completed.

What is the national average? A 2021 review in Pain Physician[64] showed that 30–50% of patients who get facet injections end up with radiofrequency ablation. After a first successful epidural, 30–40% of patients required a repeat epidural at 3–6 months, and 40–60% required a repeat by one year.[65] A 2024 observation on X/twitter (@ PainPhysicianMD) suggests that two-thirds of patients with initial success from an epidural will require regular epidurals every six to nine months to keep the pain at bay. Our results showed a radiofrequency rate of just under 7% and a repeat epidural rate of 14% at 18 months. Our results after that point are even better as it is rare to have a patient who has been through our program return with pain.

Why are our results so good? The first reason is an accurate diagnosis. This is why we have spent time deconstructing your beliefs and describing your Body Guitar. You cannot make a diagnosis from a book. Presentation of possibilities is all I can do. Finding a doctor to make this diagnosis is hard, but it was impossible before you read this last chapter. Healthcare professionals will recognize that I am calling for a complete change in this diagnosis process. A shift from disc and nerve pain only to a complex diagnosis that includes both musculoskeletal and disc/nerve. We have numerous patients that have joint pain with all the progressive spread to other areas described above AND a symptomatic disc bulge with nerve pain. This is a very complex diagnosis with a very complex treatment plan. One that would never be approached with the current algorithm. This change needs to happen as the next part of the book is about rehab. Rehab is the second reason we have good results. Rehab cannot be started until an accurate diagnosis is made and pain is reduced. This next chapter begins the second part of the book, which is how our body gets back in tune. The first part of the book was a revolution in diagnosis, and the second part will be a revolution in lumbar stability and rehabilitation. It is the Tune Me Method.

Congratulations on starting your own revolution.

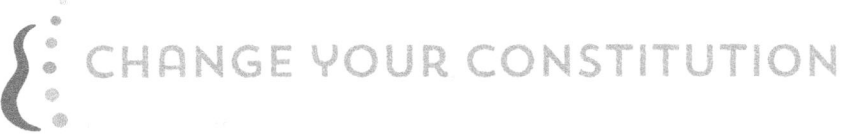 CHANGE YOUR CONSTITUTION

Your time is limited, so don't waste it living someone else's life. Don't be trapped by dogma, which is living with the results of other people's thinking. Don't let the noise of others' opinions drown out your own inner voice. And most important, have the courage to follow your heart and intuition—they somehow already know what you truly want to become. Everything else is secondary.

—Steve Jobs, 2005

The previous chapter was significant because we looked at how one back pain problem can develop into multiple problems. That chapter destroys the current treatment algorithm for back pain. You cannot have an algorithm that treats one thing at a time and uses the results of that treatment to make a diagnosis when the back doesn't work that way. The medical establishment's manner of coping with this is like one big game of whack-a-mole. The problem is that the number of moles is increasing as the establishment tries to get one mole at a time. The only way to stop the progression is to treat multiple problems at once (last chapter) and then stabilize the spine (next chapter). Before that, we have to address how the body resists your return to normal and why. (This chapter)

Our body will go through layers of unconscious adjustments to compensate for Bracing Muscle weakness and stabilize the lower back at all costs. Though these adjustments allow us to remain upright, over the long term, they warp your Body Guitar and lead to more problems, including disc breakdown, sacroiliac joint inflammation and pain, joint immobility, and a whole host of other potential problems.

The difficulty in getting the Bracing Muscles firing again and getting joint mobility and String Muscle length back is why we call this "change your constitution." If you have back pain, you must make some serious changes. You are not going to get better without a conscious decision every day to get this strength and mobility back. Because when you develop pain and the Bracing Muscles weaken, your constitution changes.

> **For forty or fifty years now, the medical establishment has been treating chronic low back pain by simply treating the pain.**

For forty or fifty years now, the medical establishment has been treating chronic low back pain by simply treating the pain. Treating the pain is necessary but insufficient. Medical advancements continue to deliver more and better treatments for pain, but these treatments don't fix the underlying causes of back pain, nor do they arrest its progression.

I want to be clear: Treating the pain is absolutely necessary, but doing so without addressing muscle weakness and all the compensations sets the patient up for the return of pain. For this reason, treating the pain as the medical establishment currently does can actually be detrimental to the patient. It results in patients getting short-term relief, then having to return for more and more treatments that become less and less effective. We have to begin to treat low back pain with the idea that we are creating time to unravel all the issues. In the last chapter, we discussed the cascade of pain, weakness, inhibition, muscle tightness, and compensation. As we begin to try to unravel these problems, we have to understand more of what holds us back. Let us start with the different kinds of muscles so that you can understand that each job is different and how long strengthening could take.

ACTION MUSCLES

When we think of muscles, we primarily think of Action Muscles. These are the muscles that move us. Action Muscles can be either of two kinds of muscles: ballistic and endurance muscles. Ballistic muscles are often called white muscles (also called Type II muscles) because they appear somewhat white by sight (when the skin is not covering them). They look relatively white because the blood flow to the individual muscle fibers is limited. These muscles store energy in the muscle like a warehouse. White muscles contract, until the stores are depleted, then we quit moving.[1]

We can develop and keep ballistic muscles strong by working them out in the gym through resistance training, such as weight-lifting, which breaks them down and then builds them back bigger and stronger. The stress caused by the workout tells the body that we need more of this muscle, and we adapt by making it bigger and more able to withstand the same load next time.

Bodybuilders focus on ballistic muscles, as do many athletes. These muscles are relatively easy to work out, and most people understand how to do so: hit the gym and the muscles get bigger and stronger. For example, doing bicep curls will strengthen the ballistic muscles in your upper arm. After about six weeks of such strengthening exercises, most people will see a significant and noticeable improvement in their ballistic muscles in the form of increased strength and size.[2] Conversely, taking a few weeks off will not likely result in a rapid loss of any gains.[3] The small amount of atrophy (muscle shrinkage) that occurs during the break can be rapidly reversed. In fact, the lost size is much easier to recover than it was to gain in the first place.[4]

The endurance muscles, on the other hand, tend not to gain size or much strength, only endurance[5] (hence the name). Endurance muscles are often called red muscles (also called Type I muscles) because, under the skin, these muscles appear redder than the ballistic muscles.[1] The red color is due to the significant blood flow through these small muscle fibers.[6] These muscles don't store much energy, but because of the constant inflow of energy from the blood, they can work much longer than the ballistic muscles.[7]

Gaining muscle endurance is not a fast or easy task.[8] Working out a red muscle involves increasing the blood flow to the muscle.[9] You cannot strengthen them by pumping iron—you must "pump blood." The goal is to get the muscles to build more blood vessels for greater endurance.[10] These are small vessels that go to the individual muscle fibers. Achieving this increased blood flow takes six months or longer.[11]

This is why marathon runners take so long to prepare for races. If you have ever tried to prepare for a marathon in six weeks, you know it is impossible. Without good blood flow, the body cannot resupply the nutrients and energy the muscles need. Six weeks is not long enough to build out these blood vessels for the rigors of a marathon.

When runners take a couple of weeks off, they see a more significant decline in endurance than a weightlifter, who only trains ballistic muscles, would experience.[3] This is because the blood vessels in the endurance muscles that runners depend upon are so small that they collapse and break down when not in use.[12] After a long interval, you'll have to start over with your training.[13]

How quickly do endurance muscles lose their endurance? In a study[14] done on rats, researchers suspended the rats' hindlegs for seven days. When the casts were removed, researchers found that the plantaris muscle (ballistic) lost little strength, but their soleus muscle (endurance) lost 40% of both size and strength in just seven days. In human bedrest studies, the same type of results have been seen in one week with endurance muscle atrophy and strength loss of up to 30% while ballistic muscle strength declines less than 10%.[15] This clearly shows that endurance muscles weaken much faster than ballistic muscles.

The Action Muscles in your body can be ballistic, endurance, or both. Also, if you are a bodybuilder and decide to change everything and become a marathoner, as you train, your muscles can change from white to red or vice versa.[16] Genetics play a role, too.[17] Some people are red/endurance muscle dominant and will never be hulking bodybuilders, but that doesn't mean they can't build up their white/ballistic muscles. Some people are ballistic dominant and will never be great distance runners, but that doesn't mean they cannot build their endurance muscles.[18] Understanding what endurance Action Muscles are is important in the care of low back pain because all String Muscles are endurance Action Muscles.

Ballistic Action Muscles	Endurance Action Muscles
Composed of "white" muscles	Composed of "red" muscles
Gain strength by "pumping iron"	Gain endurance by "pumping blood"
Can strengthen in weeks	Takes many months to strengthen
Weaken slowly when not used	Weaken rapidly when not used

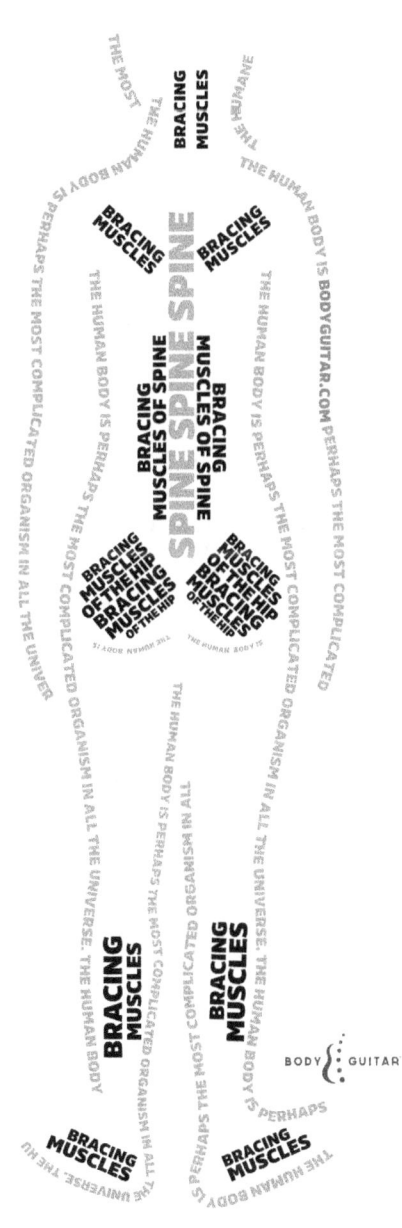

BRACING MUSCLES

Throughout the book, I have referred to the Bracing Muscles of the body that provide the baseline stability for movement *(See illustration above).* There are six sets of Bracing Muscles in the body:

1. Deep muscles of the neck Bracing Muscles
2. Base of the scapula Bracing Muscles
3. Bracing Muscles of the lumbar spine
4. Bracing Muscles of the hip
5. Ankle/knee Bracing Muscle (soleus)
6. Small Bracing Muscles of the foot

Why have I been highlighting the Bracing Muscles and why are they so different? There are many reasons, but the first difference is that Bracing Muscles are high-tone muscles that are always pulling. They can be stretched, but their natural state is short, like a spring. If your bicep was a Bracing Muscle, you would spend all of your time with your elbows bent, hands on your chest just under your chin. You could have something or someone straighten your arm, but it would snap back into the shortened state when released.

All Bracing Muscles have stretch receptors. This means that while they contract when short, they can be stretched, and this stretch provides feedback to the brain about where the body is in space.[19] This is called proprioception. If you are walking through your living room in the dark, you feel around until you touch the couch, which orients you to the room, and you can then navigate the room more easily. When we move in a direction with any muscles with stretch receptors, like the Bracing Muscles, they orient us to where our body parts are in relation to the rest of the body.[20] This includes rebalancing when walking down steps, not falling over when bending over to pick something up, or knowing when to release the ball when throwing to hit where you are aiming. Bracing Muscles are postural and they resist motion when an external force is applied by using these stretch receptors.

Unlike the Action Muscles, the Bracing Muscles can't be strengthened with motion. You can't just start running or lifting weights to strengthen the Bracing Muscles. You have to remove anything that would inhibit the muscles (pain, String Muscle contraction, positions that stretch the Bracing Muscle) and then do motions that would be resisted by the Bracing Muscles.[21] Postural motions as the Bracing Muscles attempt to resist the change in posture. Another problem with Bracing Muscles is that it is difficult to consciously know when you fatigue these muscles and begin to compensate.[22] We seamlessly have String Muscles take over when necessary, and one has to become well-versed in understanding when the Bracing Muscle fatigues and what compensation looks like.[23]

The next difference is that Bracing Muscles can NEVER be anything except red/endurance muscles.[24] The small muscles of the foot are Bracing Muscles, and no matter how hard or how long you work these muscles, you will never work your way into a larger shoe size because your foot has gotten jacked. The same goes for the Bracing Muscles in your neck. These muscles brace your neck, and if they were ever able to grow in size, they could impede your breathing. Also, the Bracing Muscles are meant to stabilize us all day long, and this requires that they be endurance muscles. The negative of this is that Bracing Muscles, like the endurance Action Muscles, when they stop firing, they weaken quickly and take a long time to return to form. So, our most important postural muscles can lose blood flow rapidly and take months to build back strength.

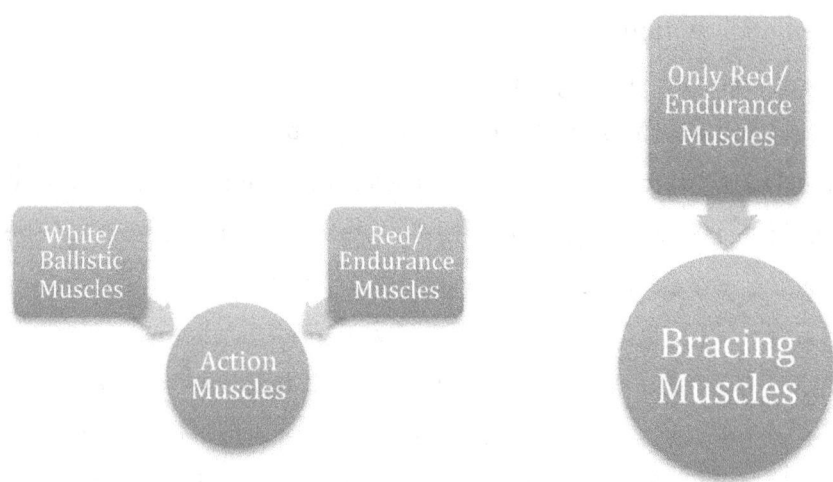

This same effect has been documented in research studies[25] observing the effect of weightlessness in outer space on the different muscle groups. Seven astronauts were tested for muscle strength before and after a two-week trip into space. Researchers found that, during those two weeks in space, Action Muscle strength had decreased by 5% in the arms and 7% in the legs, while strength in the postural muscles of the spine decreased by up to 30%. The astronauts continued to exercise daily while in space, but they weren't using their Bracing Muscles while weightless because the body didn't need to be stabilized against gravity.

If any other part of the body had lost up to 30% of its strength in that time, you would have heard about it on the prime-time news. There would have been comical reports welcoming back the astronauts but lamenting the fact that they could no longer walk. "Look at them trying to lift the escape hatch with their noodle arms," spectators might say. Bracing Muscle weakness is not so visibly apparent, but as we have seen, it can have devastating effects if strength is not restored. In fact, astronauts who return from prolonged space time are found to have 4.5 times the rate of lumbar disc bulges in the first year back compared to age matched people.[26]

It should be becoming more clear how hard it is to keep the Bracing Muscles, which again are always entirely made up of spring-like endurance muscles, strong and working well. They weaken quickly, and it is hard for them to get back in shape. They cannot be worked out in the gym—they can only be strengthened by the body creating more blood vessels, and the body will only do this when the muscles are in constant use. The trouble is that String Muscles take over, causing pain, breath holding, and locking us into a cycle where the Bracing Muscles don't get used and never regain lost strength.

Action Muscles	Bracing Muscles
Ballistic or endurance	Endurance muscles
Short or long recovery based on muscle type	Long recovery
Move to strengthen	No moving to strengthen
Easy to recognize a fatigued muscle	Hard to recognize a fatigued muscle
Don't compensate when muscle fatigues	Compensate when muscle fatigues
Recover by getting back to normal activities	Can't recover by return to normal activities
Visual and measurable improvement	No visual improvement & difficult to measure improvement
Work less well when hurt, but still work	Muscle inhibited with pain or increased sympathetic tone
Shorten when contracting (pulley)	Always short, allow lengthening (spring)
Move against external force	Resist movement against external force
Can turn on or off	Always on, but can be inhibited

Let us begin to go through why and how the body uses String

Muscles and why the balance between them and Bracing Muscles are so important.

LUMBAR STABILITY

Before we can define the problems that back pain causes, we must establish what is normal stability in the spine. There are three levels of stability, ranging from very relaxed and mobile to very tight and immobile, depending on our daily needs.

1. Bracing Muscle/Postural/String Muscles
2. Core Muscles
3. Bearing down

The lowest level is thoughtless and is the most important. It is also the foundation upon which each of the other levels is built. This lowest level includes two distinct muscle groups that provide stability based on two separate and defined modes in the body.

Our **Central Nervous System** is made up of the brain and spinal cord. Our **Peripheral Nervous System** is the other nerves in your body. These peripheral nerves can be motor nerves, which cause muscles to move. They can be sensory nerves, carrying information about all our five senses from the body to the brain. (Touch, smell, taste, hearing, and sight.) Or they can be autonomic nerves, which function unconsciously. Autonomic nerves are always working, managing subconscious processes that keep us alive, including heart rate, blood pressure, food digestion, and breathing. These autonomic nerves interact with the brain, both sending and receiving messages from the brain. Because it involves the brain, spinal cord, and sensory and motor nerves all working in the unconscious, we often call this whole system the **Autonomic Nervous System.**

This autonomic nervous system has three distinct jobs. The first is the **Enteric Nervous System**, which is how the body digests food and is not part of our discussion. The next two are the **Sympathetic** and **Parasympathetic Nervous Systems** or divisions of the autonomic nervous system.[27] These two systems are critical in lumbar stability because each uses entirely different muscle groups to stabilize the spine at the lowest level.

PARASYMPATHETIC NERVOUS SYSTEM

The parasympathetic nervous system is often called the "rest-and-digest" or "feed-and-breed" system. This system is in use when we need to eat, relax, sleep, along with other functions that counteract the sympathetic nervous system. This is the mode in which our Bracing Muscles are being used to create stability throughout the body.

To reiterate from the last chapter, in the lumbar spine, these Bracing Muscles that create a neutral pelvis are the transverse abdominis on the front of the pelvis and the spinae erector muscles on the back of the pelvis. The third muscle is the multifidus, high-tone muscles that hold the spine in neutral. Like all Bracing Muscles, these muscles are like springs that allow motion but snap back into place. *(See illustration.)*

BRACING MUSCLES OF SPINE

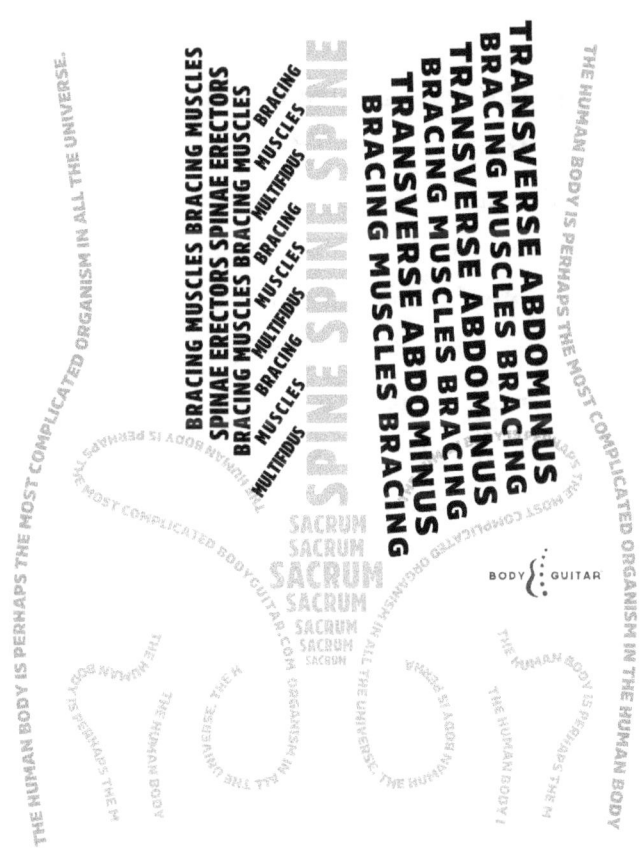

In fact, all Bracing Muscles throughout the body are parasympathetic muscles.[28] We must be in a relaxed state to use them fully.[29,30] The Bracing Muscles are strongest when you are relaxed, because the String Muscles are not contracting and the Bracing Muscles are able to be in their shortest, most active position.

SYMPATHETIC NERVOUS SYSTEM

The Sympathetic Nervous System is much more recognizable to most people. It is the "fight-or-flight" response and is active when we are stressed or in danger. Your heart rate increases, pupils dilate, and breathing increases. Your body is ready for action.

To reiterate from the last chapter, in the lumbar spine, the String Muscles used in this sympathetic stability are the psoas, iliacus, and quadratus lumborum. The psoas is in front of the vertebrae and runs from hip to diaphragm, and the iliacus and quadratus lumborum are behind the vertebrae from the hip and pelvis to the diaphragm. *(See illustration next page.)*

These muscles contract when we are in "fight-or-flight,"[31] and in this state they lock the diaphragm and pelvic floor in place along with pull hard on the femur, preparing the body for sprinting. When not in "fight-or-flight" they work at a low level to balance the body in stability with the Bracing Muscles both pulling in opposite directions, creating stability. Because these muscles are a mix of ballistic and endurance muscles rather than the Bracing Muscles which are all endurance, they fatigue differently.[32] They are, in part, endurance Action Muscles, and as such, they fatigue, spasm, and chronically tighten if asked to work beyond their capabilities.

STRING MUSCLES OF SPINE

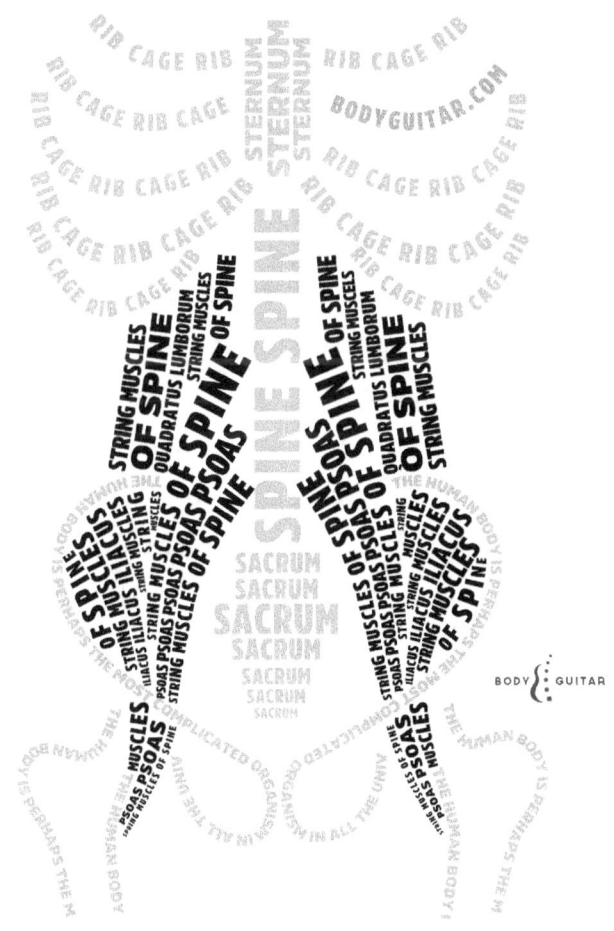

NORMAL STABILITY BALANCE

Dr. Manohar M. Panjabi's model of spine stability,[33] introduced in 1992, describes three independent subsystems that work together to maintain spinal stability. The passive subsystem made up of vertebrae, discs, ligaments and joints. The active subsystem made up of spinal muscles and tendons, and the nervous control subsystem made up of nerves, central nervous system and peripheral mechano-receptors. His description of this stability has been the framework that all subsequent theories have built upon and mine is no different.

Stuart McGill, in 2002, produced a book called *Low Back Disorders: Evidence Based Prevention and Rehabilitation*, in which he described his guy wire system. Where he addresses the active subsystem and likens the core muscles to a guy wire system, similar to cables that stabilize a structure like a radio tower.

The biopsychosocial model for back pain is a comprehensive framework that explains low back pain as a multifaceted condition influenced by biological, psychological and social factors. Basically meaning that it is influenced by the world around us and how it affect us internally, rather than just the physical or structural issues. Proposed by George Engel in 1977 and adapted for pain by researchers like Gordon Waddell, this model is in direct contrast with the traditional biomedical model, which focuses on physical pathology only. The Body Guitar theory I propose in this book, brings each of these models together. It builds on the shoulders of giants.

We have an amazing interplay of parasympathetic Bracing Muscle stability combined with sympathetic String Muscles and intra-abdominal pressure that creates thoughtless stability in the spine, providing different levels of stability when we need it, inhibiting each other to maximize their ability to provide stability while allowing different levels of mobility. Each augments our capability to move and live active lives.

By introducing Bracing Muscles, I am able to create a passive muscle group that shifts the guy wire theory slightly and builds upon it. The Bracing Muscles are like the wood of the guitar and provide significant small segment stability in a passive sense but powerful as the multifidus are considered our strongest lumbar stabilizers. The String Muscles are like the strings of the guitar creating active large segment stability. Together they create significant stability and allow both modes to work in concert.

On top of each of these two different modes of baseline static stability, we add a second level of stability by core muscles. The stronger our core muscles are, the more dynamic stability we create and they allow us to be stable through increasing ranges of motion.[34] Core muscle strength is the guy wire system that Stuart McGill proposes and instead of contradicting him, I am merely adding to it with the Body Guitar Theory. These guy wires must be thoughtless tone also, but additive to the postural stability. Weakness in core muscles leads to a potential back injury during motion and strength in core muscles protects the spine even in an unbalanced Body Guitar. (Do not

confuse core strength tone, which should be effortless, with holding your stomach in or actively rolling your pelvis under you.) Then
on top of that, we can add bearing down. When we bear down, we
breath hold to create maximal stability to protect the spine when
lifting something heavy, defecating, or birthing a child.[35] The breath-
holding that happens with String Muscles is different, as bearing
down is a *contraction* of the **pelvic floor and diaphragm** to increase
intra-abdominal pressure, which locks the String Muscles in place.
Sympathetic breath-holding is a *contraction* of the **String Muscles**,
which locks the pelvic floor and diaphragm in place and increases
intra-abdominal pressure. This may seem like a small difference, but
it is monumental.[36]

Remember from the last chapter that back pain inhibits the Bracing Muscles of the lumbar spine as these muscles would pull the
facets together. If the facets hurt or a disc is irritating nerves in the
lumbar spine, the Bracing Muscles are making this pain worse, so
they are inhibited. Then, when the sympathetic String Muscles start
to pull the spine into a less painful position, the String Muscles also
inhibit the Bracing Muscles. When the String Muscles fatigue, and
we rest in positions that allow the spine to be bent forward, these
positions also inhibit the Bracing Muscles. What we are left with is
complete or almost complete inhibition of the parasympathetic
Bracing Muscles[37] and complete or almost complete reliance on the
sympathetic String Muscles.[38] I have called these sympathetic "fight-
or-flight" muscles. But what if we are not under stress or in

"fight-or-flight"? By using these muscles throughout the day, does our body perceive these positions and create all the signs and symptoms of "fight-or-flight"? In sympathetic overload in people without back pain, they chest breathe, they have increased inflammation to prepare for injury or deal with injury, they begin to show all the same signs as someone with chronic back pain. With low back pain does our cortisol rise? Do our pupils dilate? Do our bowels slow? Does inflammation increase just because of muscle firing?[39] We know our breathing changes as we go from abdominal and chest breathing to just chest breathing because of how the muscles lock the diaphragm and pelvis, but has back pain shifted us into chronic sympathetic overload?[40] I believe so, and in my chronic low back pain patients, they show every sign of sympathetic overload.

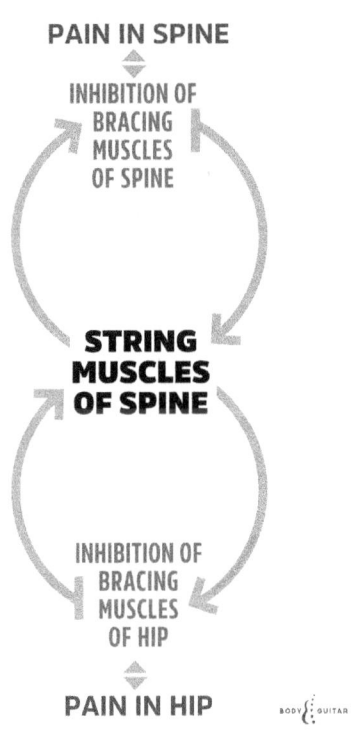

This sympathetic overload is not the balance of string and Bracing Muscles that should be making up a significant majority of a person's day. It is the sprinting "fight-or-flight" mode that is supposed to be rare during the day. Chest breathing, buttock clamped, elevated heart rate all day that is also causing long-term weakening of the Bracing Muscles and creating a situation where the lumbar spine stability is completely out of balance. The understanding of the muscles being parasympathetic and sympathetic also begins to bring the biopsychosocial model from contrasting the biomedical model to augmenting each other.

Once you remember the inhibition of the Bracing Muscles of the hip and how these weakened hip muscles cause a cycle of pain, weakness, spasm, breath-holding, and inhibition, you begin to realize how deep of a hole the chronic back pain patient is in and the generations of back pain without a cure begin to make sense.

Imagine you get on a bus, and there is nowhere to sit, so you stand in the aisle holding on to the handrail above you. Before the bus moves, you hear your phone ding that there is a message, so you let go of the railing and just stand with your feet apart. Then the bus starts to move, and you stand swaying as the bus rambles down the road and through the twists and turns of the city. Two people are standing next to each other, one with no back pain, using Bracing Muscles of the spine, String Muscles, and core strength to seamlessly and thoughtlessly stabilize themself. The other has back pain and is using only String Muscles and core strength to hold themselves stable, butt cheeks clamped, chest breathing as the diaphragm is locked. This back pain sufferer would fatigue these String Muscles and cause irritation of their back for the rest of the day.

Now, imagine there is a third person on the bus. This person had back pain but got treatment. The problem is that even a few weeks of back pain can lead to weakness and atrophy of the Bracing Muscles of the spine and hips. Because the Bracing Muscles act like springs, it is difficult to notice when a spring stops doing its job. But the nervous system knows and switches to the String Muscles to keep the body stable. This third person is also standing with butt cheeks clamped, chest breathing in "fight-or-flight" mode without knowing that they have no balance between their parasympathetic and sympathetic muscles. This third person thinks they have cured their back pain, but they have only treated the symptoms, not the disruption of their entire stability system.

In an acoustic guitar, if the wood struts inside the guitar lose their glue or crack and are not doing their job to stabilize the guitar, it is often difficult to recognize. This out-of-tune guitar is tuned by adjusting the strings to the right key, and the instrument sounds great—for a few hours or a few days. Then the strings have to be tightened again. And again. As the strings get tighter and tighter, the guitar is breaking down inside incrementally. Often, this happens so slowly that it is hard to recognize unless one carefully examines the guitar. A luthier is an expert guitar repairman. As I have explained before, we have proceduralists. We need diagnosticians, and more than that, we need Body Guitar luthiers. Because your Body Guitar is not just out-of-tune, it is weak on the inside and warped.

The cycle of pain is the real cause of why people get back pain and stay in pain. Just getting out of pain is only half the battle. You have to get out of pain, stop compensating with String Muscles, and build not just strength, but tone in your Bracing Muscles of the spine and hip, so that we can get back to the beautiful interplay of the two modes of static stability playing off each other. It is not an easy task, but it has led to a complete overhaul of the Tune Me system. Let us go through some more of the unconscious physical findings of the nervous control subsystem that are present in all adults and every chronic pain patient.

STABILITY GAP

Imagine if I laid out an agility ladder and had a bunch of 10-year-olds run through, doing intricate footwork between the ropes. You would be surprised at how uncoordinated most of them would look. This is because as a person becomes more stable, they can become more coordinated.[41] Stability is necessary for coordination to develop, and 10-year-olds are often growing so fast that their stability is still catching up.[42] Between the ages of 10 and 20, stability often greatly improves, and many of us are at the most coordinated points in our lives in our 20s.[43] As we age or get injured and become less stable,[44] you would expect that this loss of stability would lead to a loss of coordination that follows exactly as coordination was gained but in reverse.[45] But this is not what happens. Because we have developed neural patterns of motion with our coordination, when we lose our stability, we actually maintain these neural patterns. We are able to complete many coordinated movements.[46]

Think of an aged basketball player who, when younger, spent many years trying to perfect his layup. Then, years later, after having not done a layup for decades, he is able to complete a layup with perfect form after three or four tries. This is not because he still has stability but because he has neural patterns of coordination that took years to develop and are still present. But there is a gap between his coordination and Bracing Muscle stability. To protect him from his own instability, his body has to come up with other ways to create stability. We call this gap a Stability Gap. String Muscles will become chronically shorter to mimic stability. Joints and joint capsules tighten to mimic stability. Fascia tightens to mimic stability. A breath-holding compensation begins to mimic stability. Eventually, as the joints do not tolerate instability, they will begin to build bone to stabilize the joint. We call this bone growth arthritis. All of these problems need to be unwound as the unsuspecting back pain patient, who is feeling better, has no idea what they are fighting to overcome each of these problems.

MUSCLE COMPENSATION

Each of the Bracing Muscles has very specific String Muscles that will tighten to mimic stability. These attempt to stabilize you when the Bracing Muscles stop firing or fatigue, though you can't easily tell when your String Muscles take over. If you are running a race and your Action Muscles fatigue, you quit running. If you are going through the day and your Bracing Muscles fatigue, no one stops and says, "I must stop for the day. My Bracing Muscles just fatigued, and I began overusing my String Muscles to compensate." Nope. You keep going, completely unaware of the compensation. The same goes for when we try to strengthen Bracing Muscles. Not only do they strengthen like endurance muscles (very slowly over six or more months), but as we get to the point of stressing the muscles enough to demand the body to make more blood vessels, we also begin to overuse String Muscles to make up for their fatigue.

Bracing Muscle	String Muscle
Small muscles of Foot	Heel Cord, Gastrocnemius, Plantar Fascia
Soleus	Gastrocnemius, Hamstring, Anterior Tibialis
Bracing Muscles of Hip	String Muscles of Lumbar Spine, Hamstring and Quad Muscles, Piriformis
Bracing Muscles of Spine	String Muscles of Lumbar Spine, Hamstring
Lower Scapula	Rhomboid Minor, Pec Minor, Posterior Neck Muscles, Sternocleidomastoid Muscle
Deep Muscles of Neck	Posterior Neck Muscles, Sternocleidomastoid Muscle, Scalene Muscles

This sequence allows our Bracing Muscles to weaken indefinitely. No other type of muscle in your body has this type of complete and seamless muscle compensation. This is why you can recover from an action injury by returning to normal activities, but Bracing Muscles need so much more to recover.

These String Muscles don't just tighten to compensate; they increase their tone to provide stability. The problem is that they were not made for constant contraction. Bracing and core muscles are designed to be spring-like and tight. They allow motion, then snap back into their shortened, natural state. String Muscles are more like a motor that can only pull.[47] To push, an opposing muscle has to pull while the first relaxes. This means that while a spring creates tone almost without work, the pull motor has to be red lining to work all day. So, a tight Bracing Muscle is healthy, but if a String Muscle is tight and trying to do the job of a spring, it will fatigue, spasm, and essentially scream for relief. When patients tell me certain String Muscles are always tight or can never really stretch, this helps me identify which Bracing Muscles are weak.

One of the problems is when we have built back our stability but can't get the nervous system to let our muscles stretch. This becomes a reprogramming problem where the brain is trying to protect us as it has for years, and we need to convince it to back off.

When a patient begins physical therapy, I tell them that the physical therapist's job is to recognize when you begin to compensate. Their exercises are then set to avoid compensation and to teach patients when they are compensating. Patients ask if they really need to go to therapy as they can just look exercises up online. My response is always directed towards this compensation.

FASCIA AND NEURAL TIGHTNESS

Besides parasympathetic and sympathetic muscle compensation in a cycle, the central nervous system also senses the outside world and forces our bodies to compensate. The nerves, which provide input to both the muscles and fascia, play a role in providing stability.[48] The fascia is a thin layer of tissue that covers individual muscles and allows the muscles to slide on each other. It also surrounds our organs and even surrounds nerves.[49] It appears to be innervated itself, and it seems to play a part in the nervous system's stabilizing process.[50] We believe this because of how our body reacts to motion and our attempts to regain flexibility.

Have you ever tried to squat while keeping both feet flat on the floor? Some people can do this easily; we will get to those people, but most cannot. If you cannot, try it again while holding on to something stable. Why are many people now able to do it or at least do it much better? Because our brain feels more stable and allows better motion.[51] When we put patients to sleep before surgery, their nervous system is sedated, and their flexibility is greatly improved.[52] Why would our nervous system create muscle tightness that does not seem related to actual muscle being tight, but the body using muscle tightness to create stability? Because stability is so vitally important.[53] Suppose you try to create flexibility in the heel cord, hamstring, neck, shoulders, or any of the places where the String Muscles are located, and you haven't developed strength in the associated Bracing Muscles. In that case, the fascia and the nervous system will fight you.[54] If you are naturally flexible or can overcome this protective system, the body will be forced to protect you in other ways that we will get to in the arthritis section below.

Lorimer Moseley, a professor of clinical neuroscience at the University of South Australia, tells an illustrative story in his book, "Explain Pain."[55] He was in the bush one day camping, and while walking, he felt a scratch on the outside of his left leg. His nervous system took in the information from the scratch and what his eyes could see around him and determined that he was in no danger. This all happened in less than a second as his leg kicked out slightly to push away whatever scratched him. He continued to the river and washed off, got out, and collapsed. He'd been bitten by an Eastern Brown snake, the second most poisonous land snake in Australia. He almost died and had leg swelling for months, requiring rehab. Almost a year later, he was walking in the bush again and had a scratch on the same part of his left leg. This time, his nervous system sent the information to the brain, and the brain remembered his past snake bite and went into protection mode, creating excruciating pain that dropped him to his knees. His leg may have even started swelling. Someone had to pry his hands off his leg to find that he had only been scratched by a twig.

The same thing happens in a patient with long-term low back pain. This pain has disrupted their lives for a long time. Even when the pain is gone, the brain still remembers and will protect them at all costs.[56] It can make rehab difficult because our conscious mind tries to convince the unconscious mind that we are stable enough, while the unconscious mind senses the instability in our motion that the conscious mind cannot perceive. This is also affected by our inability to perceive our endurance of the Bracing Muscles consciously. As we seamlessly transition from bracing to String Muscles because of fatigue, the nervous system protects us, and we have to be patient in building back stability and endurance. We have to strengthen, stretch, and retrain the whole system.

The Gate Control Theory of Pain[57] described by Melzack and Wall in 1965 helps us understand how the brain filters some pain as insignificant and some as worth a response. The peripheral nerves send signals to the spinal cord based on injury. (Scratch on leg.) The substantia gelatinosa in the spine modulates this information, sometimes inhibiting it immediately and sometimes sending it on to the brain for a response. The brain then modulates it further through the Limbic system, and these responses can be influenced by many biopsychosocial factors that can increase or decrease the response to pain. Factors such as previous trauma or pain, stress, lack of sleep, beliefs, fears, work issues, and many others. The final determined response, if it is increased pain, can also lead to activation of the sympathetic "fight-or-flight" response and activation of the String Muscles throughout the body. So in the end, the sympathetic system can influence the brain to activate itself even more.[58]

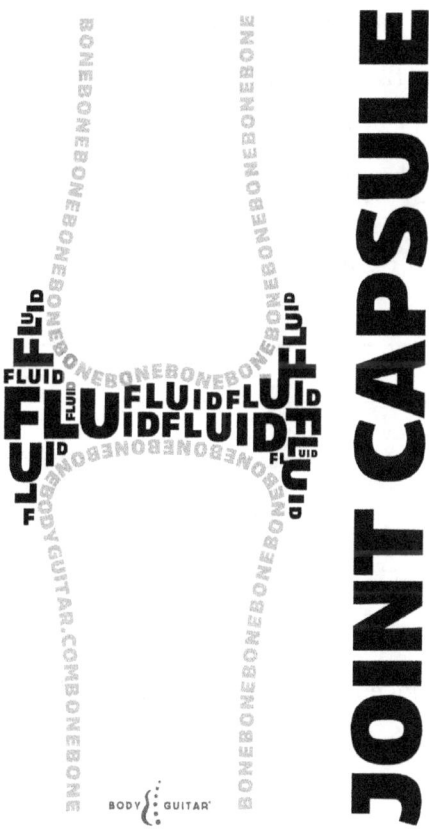

JOINT AND JOINT CAPSULE TIGHTNESS

Joints around the areas of the Bracing Muscles also tighten to compensate for Bracing Muscle weakness.[59] The joint capsule is a thin tissue that surrounds all joints in your body.[60] *(See illustration)* When it tightens, the joint moves less.[61]

In the hips, because the external rotators weaken and the knee is more likely to collapse inward, the joint capsule of the hip tightens and the joint loses mobility, thus providing stability that the muscles are not providing. Eventually, they lose the ability to sit cross-legged or turn into a golf swing, as all motion through the hip is affected.[62]

Bracing Muscle	Joint Tightness
Small muscles of Foot	Ankle
Soleus	Ankle, Knee
Bracing of Hip	Hip, Knee
Bracing of Spine	Lumbar and Thoracic Spine
Lower Scapula	Shoulder and Neck
Deep Neck	Neck

In the back, the isolated motion of the pelvis is often the first to go, as the lowest facet joints in the back develop joint tightness. As a slight forward bend is less painful for facet pain and helps create intra-spinal space for disc bulges and spinal stenosis, people often find themselves slightly bent forward.[63] Thoracic motion through the spine is often also significantly affected, and Jake McFarland, a physical therapist who works with our high-level athletes, often first starts trying to get motion here with his patients.[64]

ARTHRITIS

What happens when joint tightness, fascia and neural tightness, and tightening String Muscles are not enough to stabilize us? The joints and discs will begin to break down. The cartilage of the joint will start to wear,[65] and the discs will start to desiccate.[66] As this happens, the body will build bone to stabilize the joint or disc in a process called arthritis. Yes, arthritis happens from inflammatory disease in many cases. However, it most often occurs from a lack of stability in weight-bearing or partially weight-bearing joints.[67]

Once this happens, the condition is permanent. Active people should seek to avoid this development, though it may not be completely possible, as sometimes our motions require this extra layer of stability. As an example, a study out of Sweden[68] X-rayed elite tennis players ages 12 to 26 without back pain. Over 90% were found to have arthritis in their spine, which likely developed to protect the spine from all the twisting tennis requires.

For hypermobile individuals, the risk of arthritis is significantly higher. If a hypermobile patient loses stability, they are prone to developing arthritis and disc disease at an accelerated rate.[69] They often don't exhibit as much compensatory muscle tightness and joint capsule tightness, and while some may develop areas of neural protective tightness, it's not a guarantee. This is why I always stress to my hypermobile patients the importance of working diligently on their stability. Their unique condition sets them up for significant problems in their joints and discs.

For all patients, decreased joint motion is not just a part of aging. We have to carefully keep track of the mobility of the joints and flexibility of String Muscles and recognize that their tightness may be a sign of instability. If we don't treat the Bracing Muscle weakness early, the body will continue to try to close this Stability Gap until it becomes permanent arthritis that is much more difficult to overcome.

REHABILITATION IS NON-NEGOTIABLE

We challenge our patients to suspend their disbelief when it comes to rehab, allow us to send them to appropriate physical therapy, and use many other practitioners when it comes to retraining the whole system. Every patient is different and takes different paths, but rehab is non-negotiable. Realize also that I put the same requirements on the physical therapist. Our window is short after diagnosis and treatment. At that critical juncture, it has to be "all hands on deck."

The crucial moment for my patients is when they return for the first visit and are finally out of pain. We did everything right in diagnosis and treatment; they are always very satisfied at this stage. I then talk to them about rehab, and the whole conversation changes. They tell me they have tried physical therapy before, know all the exercises, have a great trainer, or work out all the time. It is a moment where I realize that the odds are stacked against them. Everything has to go exactly right, or I will see them back with a return of their pain in a few months. It is rare in this first round of pain that I can convince them that they are not healed and that this period of diminished pain is their opportunity to fix all the problems that months and years of pain have caused. They grasp that they have to strengthen and will try to breathe better, but everything beyond that is unnecessary as they are now fixed. When the next cycle of pain returns, they are more likely to follow my advice. If they come back. Often, though, I will see them years later when they tell me that what I did for them the first time didn't work.

"But when I saw you back, you were feeling great?"

"Yeah, but that only lasted a few months."

"But that is how long the steroids work."

"See, it didn't work."

It worked, but they didn't use the time we gave them. I try to tell them that once their pain is arrested, it is like we have turned over a sand dial, and when the sand runs out, their pain will return, unless they use this window of opportunity to reverse the chain of inter-related compensations. And get their train back on the tracks.

TUNE ME

What we have learned in this chapter is that the Bracing Muscles are easy to weaken, and when they do, they throw everything off. Remember that I told you that this is a perfect system of stability. High-tone small parasympathetic Bracing Muscles augmented by sympathetic String Muscles creating the proper amount of stability at the necessary time. Sympathetic and parasympathetic systems working together. An orchestra of muscles and intra-abdominal pressures creating stability in a poorly stabilized part of the body. When things go wrong, it becomes a complex interplay between pain, posture, breath holding, fight-or-flight, and muscle weakness.

The basic concept is that all parts of the body must work together in harmony. With a warped Body Guitar you cannot tune correctly and your back pain will continue or return.

The next chapter is about the Tune Me method, which allows you to fix your Body Guitar and to play your life song, and I can't wait to see what you can do when you are healed.

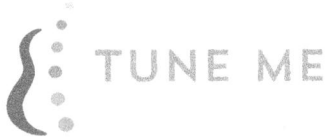

CHAPTER 6

TUNE ME

Do the difficult things while they are easy, and do the great things while they are small. A journey of a thousand miles must begin with a single step.

—Lao Tzu

Hopefully, this book has been a revelation. Your pain is more complicated than you thought, and the medical system has failed to help you recover fully. You now know the treatment algorithm is broken and flawed. The MRI is a tool, not a diagnosis, and pain causes so many downstream problems that simply getting out of pain doesn't fix you. Many well-meaning people are diligently trying to help, but they haven't devised a comprehensive plan.

This old Indian parable[1] was used by the 19th-century Hindu Saint Sri Ramakrishna Paramahamsa to describe the ill effects of dogmatism. To quote from the collection of his stories called The Ramakrishna Kathamrita:

"A number of blind men came to an elephant. Someone told

them that it was an elephant. The blind men asked, 'What is the elephant like?' as they began to touch its body. One of them said, 'It is like a pillar.' This blind man had only touched its leg. Another man said, 'The elephant is like a husking basket.' This person had only touched its ears. Similarly, he who touched its trunk or its belly talked of it differently."

In each of these cases, the blind man who touched a certain part of the elephant was completely correct in their assessment of the part that they were touching, but they did not understand the whole of the animal. This mirrors back pain treatment. When a physician treats one area at a time or relies on the MRI for a diagnosis, they are only treating what they can "touch" and not seeing the whole elephant. When a treatment protocol involves release of the psoas, it will make a difference in a patient's life temporarily, as the other parts of the problem are not understood. When a physical therapist begins to try to strengthen a muscle in a patient who is in pain, they are focused on muscle weakness and not making the muscle strength work within the whole instrument. Each of these practitioners can point to the numerous people they have helped, and, like the blind man touching the ear of the elephant, they would be correct. Yet, we need more than numerous people who are helped but continue to return for more help. We need to see the whole of the problem and treat the whole thing. By seeing each of these problems in a new light, we can then begin to think of the solution systematically. We need to understand how each part of the treatment fits together with other parts of the treatment so that we can know which part to address. You should be able to recognize what is happening to you and what the next step should be. You need to be in control of your own care, and this chapter should empower you. Because this is about you, and you are the hero of the story.

Throughout this book, I have repeatedly asked you to think of your body as a guitar. This metaphor was not chosen at random or haphazardly. Your lower back is a marvel of design, but it's not naturally stable. It's like a wobbly stack of blocks that needs a complex muscular balance to stay stable. Decades of working in and studying medicine, particularly sports medicine and pain, have made me recognize how much the lower back functions like an instrument and particularly a guitar. A guitar that can be expertly played to create the beautiful music of life.

When you have back pain, the whole instrument falls out of tune, all of the parts fall out of sync, and eventually the whole instrument becomes warped. We are supposed to have balance between the Bracing and String Muscles about 90% of the time. The remaining 10% should be balanced between resting Bracing Muscle stability and stressed String Muscle stability. In people with chronic back pain, they spend all of their time in full String Muscle contraction.

Your different parts were designed for specific tasks, and chronic pain taxes the system: String Muscles begin to dominate, Bracing

Muscles are inhibited in many ways, joints become immobile, fascia tightens down in a futile attempt to keep it all together, breath-holding takes over, and the nervous system goes into protection mode. As a result, more pain ensues. As pain causes instability, instability causes chronic pain—and the body's attempt to control instability causes both further problems and more chronic pain. Eventually even leading to String Muscle weakness as the entire lumbar spine becomes weak.

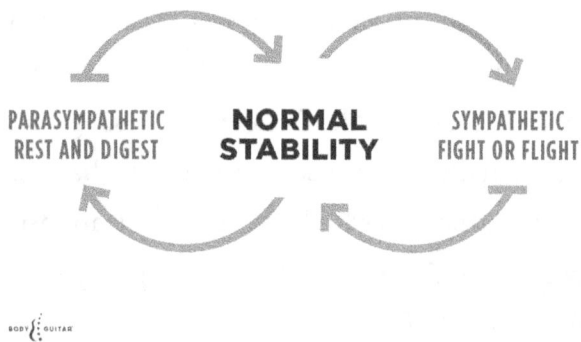

PARASYMPATHETIC   **NORMAL**   SYMPATHETIC
REST AND DIGEST   **STABILITY**   FIGHT OR FLIGHT

Your goal, after you decrease the pain, is to regain this muscle balance and stability. Understand that a treatment algorithm, an injection, or a few occasional exercises here and there will not fix your instability. It takes much more than that. You have to get everything working together again.

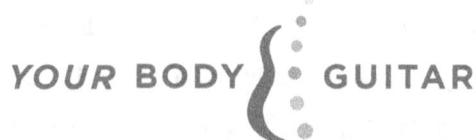

YOUR BODY ⦃ GUITAR

TUNE ME

After two decades of seeing chronic back pain patients with the same problems that were not getting better, I understood that the problem was with the way we were treating the condition. This book has so far pointed out all of the difficulties in managing chronic back pain, as well as the ways in which the medical establishment has been failing to address those issues due to institutional inertia.

It doesn't have to be this way. We have the right knowledge and right treatments—we are simply applying them without a coherent plan. If, instead of treating pain as a problem unto itself, we instead focus on the underlying weakness, instability, and resultant immobility, we can revolutionize the way we treat chronic back pain. Tune Me is not a new back pain treatment—it's about creating a whole new paradigm that frees us from the shackles of the way the medical practice has been managing chronic back pain.

To recap: Pain causes Bracing Muscle inhibition, which are the spring-like muscles that create stability and posture in a relaxed state without significant effort. Because these muscles are inhibited, we can only use the "fight-or-flight" String Muscles to create stability. Using these muscles further inhibits the Bracing Muscles. As these String Muscles are not spring-like but pull motors, they will fatigue and spasm as they red-line. We can adopt positions that relieve this fatigue and spasm, but even these positions inhibit the Bracing Muscles. As the Bracing Muscles are endurance muscles, they lose significant strength rapidly, which causes instability. Instability leads to pain, and pain then leads to more weakness in the Bracing Muscles of the spine. This leads to more problems, more pain, less mobility, and less stability. The constant contraction of the String Muscles of the spine causes inhibition of the Bracing Muscles of the hip, which creates a cycle of pain and weakness. It is a cycle that feeds on itself. Pain, instability, lack of mobility, and weakness can all result in each other. Retuning the body requires digging yourself out of the hole and inching your way backward toward good health again.

Your ultimate aim is to reclaim your stability and balance in the sympathetic and parasympathetic muscles of the spine. This is the key to your freedom of movement. We must get the sympathetic tone, which has been allowed to take over the stability of our spine, to decrease so that we can strengthen the Bracing Muscles. Working on Bracing Muscles is not about strengthening through movement (as you would with Action Muscles), but about moving to strengthen the muscles that brace you. If our sympathetic tone is high, then the String Muscles are doing all the stabilizing, and moving to strengthen ends up only strengthening the String Muscles. It's a simple concept: Our spine and body must be stable to move. We must strengthen the muscles that stabilize us. These are the Bracing Muscles and the String Muscles. By addressing these muscles, we are addressing the foundation upon which ALL motion depends. If your Bracing Muscles are not strong, your body either uses the

String Muscles or breaks down. To change this, you have to address both the String Muscle overuse and the Bracing Muscle weakness.

Some readers will be expecting actual exercises to be displayed in this chapter. I would be doing you a disservice by trying to show you exercises. That would keep you from a rehab professional, as you would believe you could do it on your own. When an amateur golfer stands on the tee and gives another golfer an assessment on what they think the other person is doing wrong, they often make things worse. They may be exactly correct in their assessment, but what they fail to realize is that in every golf swing, there are flaws and compensations. By fixing the flaw and not the compensation, the golf swing will completely fall apart. The same is true for a body. We have weaknesses and compensations. A professional golf coach and a rehab professional will address both the flaw and the compensation. Finding the right exercise for you and addressing the compensations you have made for that weakness is essential. There are some exercises in the appendix, but these are meant to take with you to a professional therapist as a starting point. They might not even be the exercise you ultimately need. Rarely, people have weak spasming String Muscles and these people have to be treated differently. The body is more complicated than a book or a set of exercises.

BREAKING IT DOWN—TUNE ME NOTE BY NOTE

Tune Me comprises six simple concepts or steps. Though simple, they are not easy, and they require time and effort to get right. The principles of Tune Me are:

1. **Tune Me: Treat the Pain First**
   You have to get your pain under control before you can stop the inhibition of the Bracing Muscles.

2. **Tune Me: Understanding Your Instrument**
   Focusing on understanding your body and what has gone wrong.

3. **Tune Me: Strumming Hand**
   Working on breaking the cycle of inhibition. This is about how to decrease the sympathetic tone.

4. **Tune Me: Fretting Hand**
   Using exercises that strengthen your Bracing Muscles.

5. **Tune Me: Feedback**
   Using correct posture, flexibility, and joint mobility to monitor your progress.

6. **Tune Me: Achieving Your 180 in 180**
   Putting in six months of work so that you can reverse the course of your chronic back pain.

Not everyone starts the journey from the same place. Some people start with no change in their sympathetic tone; most don't. Some people start with no atrophy of the Bracing Muscles of the hip; others don't. Where you start depends on your particular issues and how quickly you get into effective treatment. However, anyone with chronic back pain will have some degree of increased sympathetic tone, and certainly some degree of Bracing Muscle weakness. These issues may only become evident as we get fatigued.

It's crucial to understand that the phases of Tune Me, while presented as separate steps, are deeply interconnected. Each step is not a stand-alone process, but a part of a comprehensive whole. I'm introducing them in a specific order to guide you, but the phases will overlap. You will continue to work on all aspects of Tune Me throughout the program, and, to a lesser extent, for the rest of your life. This ongoing commitment is a key part of managing your back pain effectively.

1. Tune Me: First You Have to Treat the Pain

By now, you should understand that pain is not only the physical manifestation of problems in the back—it is also a driver of problems. Chronic back pain amplifies our sympathetic nervous system, which creates and exacerbates further back problems. Pain keeps us from using our Bracing Muscles, which causes them to become so weak that they can no longer stabilize the body.

To address chronic back pain over the long term, you have to address what is causing it: weakness, immobility, and sympathetic tone, all of which are related to instability. What patients find, however, is that they cannot address these issues while they are still in pain—so it may feel like a catch-22 to many patients caught in a cycle of treatment failure and worsening pain. Pain is what makes you weak and leads to a sympathetic overload, and until you get that pain under control, you won't be able to get better. This cycle is exacerbated by the glut of ineffective failed treatments doled out by the treatment algorithm.

So many people are treated for their pain and then wait to see if it comes back. When it comes back, they are sent to physical therapy, but they cannot do the necessary exercises while they are in pain. This becomes a waste of both time and money. Our approach is to do procedures, if necessary, to get you out of pain so that we can decrease sympathetic tone and do strengthening. Once you are out of pain, the clock has started.

One of the exams that we do after a patient returns from treatment is to see if they can gently settle into a relaxed spine position. Can you allow the lumbar spine to settle into a normal curve without your back hurting? Does it start to hurt after a while or hurt later because you were in this position? This should not be a forceful backbend, but just a slight, relaxed bend. This places the facets together and narrows the canal that the spinal cord runs through. If this position hurts, then you can't start physical therapy or decrease your sympathetic tone. Also, as you will see below, this position corrects many posture problems and really helps with the breath-holding issues. From this position, we can fire the Bracing Muscles of the spine and hip. We can use our parasympathetic system instead of the sympathetic system and begin to regain balance between these two modes. If we cannot attain this position without pain, then we cannot rehab the Bracing Muscles. If we cannot rehab the Bracing Muscles of the spine and hip, we cannot balance our stability.

You have a limited amount of time to get your Body Guitar tuned before the pain returns. You are not yet better just because the pain is gone, but this is your window of opportunity to start strengthening exercises. If you get to rehab and you find that the exercises hurt too much or cause a return of pain, you may need to go back to your doctor for more pain treatment.

All treatments for back pain can be judged by two measures: how much the pain relief will allow you to strengthen the Bracing Muscles without your back becoming too irritated to continue the exercises. The second is, can you decrease your sympathetic tone.

Some people will find that they can do the exercises at first, but over time, they will experience a return of pain that interferes with their exercises. A number of things can cause this: doing the exercises wrong (you should have a good physical therapist who can make sure that you are doing them right); or the joint is becoming irritated from the exercises, in which case you still need to go back and get more pain treatment so you can continue to do the exercises.

Some people will also find that their sympathetic tone remains high, and all their work to decrease it doesn't change this tone. Understanding your tone and learning how to recognize it also allows us to know if we need more pain treatment.

When I say to get pain treatment, I mean appropriate and effective pain treatment. You might not get that from the treatment algorithm currently in wide use. As I stated in previous chapters, you cannot just treat one thing at a time when many patients hurt in several places—too much can go wrong. If you try to treat multiple problems individually and sequentially, the first one might start hurting again by the time you finally treat the last of your problem areas. This is the problem with the current world of pain management. The ingrained algorithm doesn't work, and we are only one clinic. This will slowly change. Either medicine will change, or we will have Body Guitar Clinics throughout the world. The goal is not necessarily to have clinics everywhere; the goal is to change how back pain is treated. If that requires opening clinics throughout the world, we are committed to it.

Until that time, be ready to do whatever it takes to get the pain under control. Sometimes, that just means pain medicine or steroid injections. Other times, though, it may mean surgery or nerve ablation. If a patient consistently only gets a couple of weeks of pain relief from shots, they need more treatment. A few weeks are not enough to start getting stronger—you need months. If your problem is not related to a disc issue, most people in our clinic, around 95%, get a couple of months of pain relief from a steroid shot in their facets and sacroiliac joints, if that is consistent with their exam and diagnosis. The remaining 5%, who don't attain lasting relief from this injection, need nerve ablation. In these situations, I will burn the nerve that goes to the painful joint so that it cannot feel anything, which will buy these patients six months to two years to get in tune. In patients who do have a disc problem that is causing their pain, injections or surgery may be necessary to provide the time to retune the body.

The bottom line is this: There are two levels of baseline stability, and the parasympathetic Bracing Muscle group is the most crucial and most used because it uses basic postural muscles. You cannot utilize this level of stability when you hurt. You must get the pain under control at all costs so that you can do strengthening. After treating the pain, we have shut down one of the causes of Bracing Muscle inhibition. Those of us who treat the pain have to be like a guitar luthier. We must understand the entirety of the instrument and the whole of the problem. Otherwise, we are a blind man touching an elephant.

2. Tune Me: Understanding Your Instrument

When someone first starts playing the guitar, they learn how to take care of the instrument, what parts do what, and how to properly hold it.

The same goes for your body. When we get someone out of pain, we have to start by getting them to understand their instrument. If you have chronic back pain, your body is overtightened and breaking up from the inside. Its wood is cracking, and the shape is bowed. You need to learn about your Body Guitar and how to get it out of the mismanaged shape it is in.

This starts with a motion evaluation and physical therapy. The motion evaluation that we have developed is specifically directed toward the balance we want to create in the body. How strong are your Bracing Muscles? Which String Muscles have taken over and are too tight? Which joints have become immobile? Our motion evaluation is measurements and videos meant to assess this balance. We are working to make this available everywhere, and to understand population groups and age-matched results. The concepts are what are relevant to this section. If sympathetic tone is increased in my lower back, it has caused increased tone everywhere else in the body. If I don't recognize and identify these other areas, have I truly been healed? I only make changes to what I measure. By measuring each of these areas, and then following their improvement after physical therapy and even over the years, I can now understand my instrument and can continue to try to make measured improvements to my Body Guitar. Imagine when this becomes widespread. Someone could have a measurement done from when they were 25 and compare it to themselves at 45 after an injury. They are then aiming to regain the stability, posture, strength, and mobility that they once had. While you may realize that 45-year-olds don't move like their 25-year-old selves, we must begin to question why. By measuring each area and understanding the parasympathetic and sympathetic tone, maybe we are underselling our capabilities.

The second part of understanding your instrument is beginning physical therapy. In the hands of a good therapist, they will start by introducing you to your movements and Bracing Muscles. In the first couple of visits, you will learn about body movements that are subtle in nature. This period focuses on finding the correct muscles, not necessarily strengthening them yet. It usually involves patients lying down in a position that isolates particular Bracing Muscles of the spine and hip, and then making extremely slight movements that force the Bracing Muscles to stabilize the spine and hip.

You cannot move on to the next step until you know what contracting the Bracing Muscles feels like and how to tell if your String Muscles are helping. For some people, this is a one-visit process, and for others, it takes several visits.

I usually see people struggle with this when they are with their therapist—but as they continue to work on it at home, they show up with a much better understanding. It doesn't matter how long it takes; you must understand your instrument before progressing.

But the patient can't tell, at first, that they are using the wrong muscles. These people often come in thinking they are already strong and don't need exercises, which couldn't be further from the truth.

There are tricky parts to isolating the correct muscles. You need to know when you are stabilizing with parasympathetic Bracing Muscles of the spine and hip, and when you are stabilizing with the sympathetic String Muscles. You need an expert physical therapist to help you isolate the muscles; it is not something that you can usually do on your own. You will not be able to recognize when you are compensating in the beginning.

After isolating the muscles, you must be taught diaphragmatic breathing, good posture, and how to stretch your String Muscles and joints properly. This is also vital information about your Body Guitar that you will use for the rest of your life, so treat it as such.

Find a good physical therapist who can teach you how to understand your instrument. Getting pain relief only to do the exercises wrong is a waste of time, effort, and money. I usually won't even agree to do the pain treatment if the patient is unwilling to then go and sit down with a rehabilitation specialist who will help them isolate and work out the right muscles.

3. Tune Me: Strumming Hand

When I first started playing the guitar, I had to count out the strums. Down-down-up—up-down-up is a very common strum pattern. When playing a song, I had to repeat it to myself over and over as I played it. Then, as time went on, I got better at the strum and could do it without thinking about it. As the years have gone by while playing guitar, I can now hear a song, feel its rhythm, and reproduce that in my strumming pattern just from what sounds good. We want the same result from your Body Guitar.

In this stage, you will learn autonomic nervous system control. As stated in the last chapter, the sympathetic String Muscles take over as the dominant mode of stability when one has low back pain. We are normally supposed to have a balance between parasympathetic Bracing Muscles of the lumbar spine and sympathetic String Muscles of the lumbar spine. A little bit of country and a little bit of rock'n'roll. When we get low back pain, the inhibition of the Bracing Muscles leads to only being able to use the String Muscles for stability. Much like the "fake it until you make it" mantra that some people live by, being in a position of "fight-or-flight" and using the String Muscles of "fight-or-flight" eventually convinces our brains that we are in "fight-or-flight." We must begin to recognize the sympathetic overload so that we can counteract it before it begins to have the same effect on the neck, shoulders, calves, and feet—because it will.

When we stand with low back pain and String Muscle dominance, the String Muscles attempt to pull everything into a shortened position to keep it stable. (Think of the straps on a load in the back of a pickup truck.) As the lumbar spine is vertebrae stacked one on another, it can only shorten so far, so the String Muscles pull hard on the femur (hip bone). This inhibits the Bracing Muscles of the hip and the remaining butt muscles tighten. Don't be confused that this has something to do with standing, as the chronic back pain sufferer will lie in bed with a straight spine and the butt cheeks clamped. Then, when slouching or in a fetal position when lying down, butt cheeks are relaxed as the femur is locked in this position, and the back pain sufferer can sleep or sit with less pain. But the vertebrae are not stacked, and the String Muscles tighten into this bent-over position to provide stability. Then, when one tries to get up, they struggle as the String Muscles have to be "unratcheted" out of this bent position. Then, when they finally get the vertebrae stacked and straight, the butt muscles tighten up again. This cycle of butt clamped when spine straight, and difficulty straightening back up when bent over, is found repeatedly in back pain sufferers. Some people think that this will go away when their pain is gone, but it is a sign of what the body has done to maintain stability. It is a red flag waving, telling us we have high sympathetic tone. Just because we have treated a patient's pain does not mean that we have fixed this sympathetic tone.

Once we decrease back pain, to decrease this sympathetic tone, we have to get the diaphragm moving again. When the diaphragm moves, this will relax the String Muscles, and vice versa. When we decrease pain, we have to realize that our continued breath-holding causes inhibition of the Bracing Muscles we need for stability.

When we get out of pain, we don't just stop breath-holding, as we have new learned patterns of motion. Also, remember that the breath-holding inhibits both the Bracing Muscles of the spine and those of the hip. This means that the weakness leads to breath-holding and the breath-holding keeps you weak. To escape this trap, you have to consciously catch yourself breath-holding and force your diaphragm to move again. Concentrate on getting your back into that relaxed spine position we discussed earlier. By getting into this position, your ability to thoughtlessly abdominal breathe increases exponentially.

This is harder than you think. You are not consciously holding these muscles tight or breath-holding. It is all happening at an unconscious level and has been for months and years. And you are trapped in weakness because of this unconscious protection.

Patients will find themselves working on this particular skill for much longer than they ever expected. One method for paying attention to the unconscious was given to me by psychologist Jim Lemons, who said that he will have patients who are trying to disrupt old patterns place yellow sticky notes all over in random places around their house, car, and place of work. Every time they see one of these yellow squares, they focus on the prescribed new action or thought. In this case, abdominal breathing and relaxing the spine. Then, as the notes begin to fall, he has them find anything yellow they see as their new reminder.

One of our other tools in breaking this cycle is using any of the modalities that affect the psoas. Remember in Chapter 4 when I went through how all the common treatments for back pain involved getting the psoas to relax. I was not trying to degrade these treatments, but merely suggesting that these were a blind man touching an elephant. Their use and effectiveness are undeniable, but they must be used with the whole plan in mind. This is their place in helping us to decrease sympathetic tone.

BODY GUITAR

As we begin to understand that this balance between parasympathetic and sympathetic tone is what is happening in low back pain, we must also be aware of other contributors to sympathetic tone. "Fight-or-flight" leads to, among other things, inflammation.[2] In reverse, inflammation eventually leads to a state of "fight-or-flight."[3] If we hope to decrease inflammation and, in turn, decrease the sympathetic tone in our bodies, we need to improve the environment that our bodies exist in. We have to understand that the stress that our daily lives create shows up in our bodies. We live, eat, sleep, etc., in a fashion that sets us up for sympathetic overload because we spend most of our day in "fight-or-flight" mode.

The world of pain management has adopted a biopsychosocial model of treatment. Which really means that they are trying to decrease sympathetic tone. But they are trying to do it while someone is still in pain. This another example of a blind man touching an elephant and being completely correct on what is wrong—but not understanding the whole of the animal.

Getting our daily thirty minutes of exercise, eight hours of time in bed without phone or television, and monitoring our stress levels should be mandatory for any patient with long-term low back pain. HRV (heart rate variability) levels are an crude measure of our balance between parasympathetic and sympathetic effects on our heart rate throughout the day.[4] Many devices now measure this, and improving our understanding and working to have a higher HRV does affect our ability to combat low back pain.

Stress is a major factor in chronic pain, as pain changes our lives.

We have a pain psychologist we use who focuses on chronic pain and overcoming the protection modes that the brain has built to avoid pain. Patients even go through learning to move again, as with long-term pain, the brain has to be convinced that normal motion doesn't cause pain.[5] Cognitive behavioral therapy is an underused part of chronic pain treatment and, at its essence, is adjusting the words we tell ourselves and the behaviors we adapt when we hurt.[6]

Meditation and biofeedback are bio-hacks[7] of what our creator implanted in us as contemplative prayer. Learning to use any of these has been proven to improve our stress levels,[8] and we recommend them to our patients. We even provide classes if they are interested. Diet has been directly related to inflammation,[9] and while there are personal differences, an anti-inflammatory diet does decrease the inflammation throughout the body.[10] At our clinic, we have made this a priority and have our own nutritionist/dietitian.

Sleep is imperative, but you can't force yourself to sleep eight hours. Most adults need seven hours, and I have, throughout my life, been a six-hours/night sleeper. Lack of sleep is both a cause of inflammation and increased sympathetic tone, and a result of it.[11] Recently, I have made a commitment to spending eight hours in bed without a phone or television in an attempt to get seven hours of sleep per night. What I have found, using a device to measure my sleep, is that when I get more than one hour of deep sleep and one and a half hours of REM sleep,[12] I am rested and restored. If you don't know what I am talking about, you need to begin to look into sleep monitoring and sleep architecture.

Sunlight, as proposed by Dr. Andrew Huberman, modulates sympathetic tone primarily through its impact on circadian rhythms, hormone release, and neural circuits, with timing being a critical factor.[13]

Infection can also be a cause of inflammation in the body. I bring this up mostly because we have had patients with cavities in their teeth with festering infections that kept them from getting complete improvement in their back pain.[14]

These topics and more are vital to decreasing our sympathetic tone. I discuss all of this before learning the exercises because we must be balanced between Bracing and String Muscles if we are to strengthen correctly. If we have high sympathetic tone, then we will spend most of our time in rehab strengthening the String Muscles, as they are firing and they inhibit the Bracing Muscles. By strengthening the String Muscles, we are not getting better. So, while any guitar player will recognize that no one would learn strumming before fretting, we are unlearning faulty muscle patterns as we have developed a Stability Gap. Therefore, the process presented is going in reverse.

4. Tune Me: Fretting Hand

When playing a guitar, one of your hands must be positioned on the guitar's frets (the raised lines on the guitar neck), isolating a string or strings that make up a chord. This is a very technical part of playing a guitar. People spend a long time learning chords and how to quickly move from one chord to another until it becomes something they can do without thinking.

We want our Body Guitar to be the same way. In this stage, you will learn exercises that strengthen your Bracing Muscles. I ask my physical therapists to start most patients on a few exercises for the Bracing Muscles of the spine and a few exercises for the Bracing Muscles of the hip. Again, these are building blocks to help you learn to play your life song. Think of these exercises as the "chords" of your Body Guitar. You have to learn to play these chords individually to put together a beautiful life song. What many have found is that by strengthening one of the Bracing Muscles of the spine, the other two muscles begin to strengthen, as if the three muscles are connected and just by getting the strength back in one of them will cause all three to contract again. We find this in the multifidus stimulator where they place wires that stimulate the multifidus and discover that all the Bracing Muscles of the spine get stronger.[15] Weightlifters tell people that if they can get to a certain very heavy weight in squats and deadlift, that by strengthening the spinae erectors they can get all the Bracing Muscles of the spine stronger.[16] This is somewhat dangerous, as we don't want chronic back pain patients to start by trying to build up to very heavy weights, as they could easily get injured, but makes the point. These three Bracing Muscles of the spine seem to work together enough that strengthening one of them may lead to improved strength in each of them.

The Bracing Muscles of the hip are different. We need exercises that affect the external rotators and exercises that affect the gluteus medius and minimus. They do different jobs and work together to stabilize the femur in the joint. The physical therapist needs to find, at least, one Bracing Muscle of the spine exercise that you can do perfectly, then teach two or more Bracing Muscles of the hip exercises affecting different parts of the hip.

Over the first month or so, you need to become a master of these exercises. Learn to do them perfectly. Learn to recognize when you are using the right muscles and when you are compensating. Get comfortable with these exercises, as you will be doing them for a long time. For the most part, you will not be moved onto "more advanced" exercises. Instead, your goal is to perfect these exercises and build strength, tone, and endurance through repetitions.

As you get better at the exercises, you will increase your repetitions. You may start with ten reps and then move to twenty-five, but we never want to completely fatigue these muscles, only build more blood flow. These exercises are like the notes in a musician's chromatic scale. The chromatic scale is the building block for all songs, and musicians go over them repeatedly while training themselves. You will do the same with these exercises. Perfect practice makes perfect. Note that not everyone's exercises are the same. There are certain Bracing Muscle exercises that I do that fire the muscle perfectly, and others that I cannot keep my String Muscles from helping. One exercise is not harder than the other, but it has a completely different effect on me than it may have on another person. Your therapist should be able to find the right exercises for you.

My patients often scoff at these exercises because they are such small, isolated movements that often seem too easy. This can be hard for some people, especially young, physically strong men and women who want to hit the ground running like they are pumping iron. But pumping blood requires small movements made repetitively. Some people find that the exercises make them feel silly—they think they should be able to start with something more intense. They don't want to "waste time" doing silly little exercises.

This perspective betrays a lack of understanding about Bracing Muscles. These patients are focused on working out as they know it: being in the gym pumping iron. Working out our Bracing Muscles has nothing to do with pumping iron, though. It is circulation training. We are getting these endurance muscles redder and redder as the blood flow to them increases. You are pumping blood, not iron.

Another thing that discourages patients is the long wait to see progress. You have to learn to set aside your ego and trust in the process—if you have been in chronic pain for a long time, you almost certainly do have weak Bracing Muscles, even if your Action Muscles are strong and you can lift a lot of weight. What many people don't realize is that when Bracing Muscles are weak, these exercises can be extremely hard—if you are actually doing them correctly. If you have Bracing Muscles that fatigue easily and use them instead of the String Muscles that compensate for weak Bracing Muscles, these exercises are not easy.

WEAK BRACING MUSCLES

I had a patient a few years ago who, right before he came to see me, broke the world record at a competition in Russia for his weight class in the deadlift. He said that when he did his record-breaking lift, he had to turn his left foot out to keep his left leg from collapsing in when lifting this extraordinary weight. When I examined him, besides the facet pain he had, I also found left String Muscle spasm with resultant weakness of the Bracing Muscles of the hip. He had some of the strongest gluteus maximus muscles in the history of mankind. Still, his left Bracing Muscles of the hip were inhibited because of String Muscle tightness. It had led to weakness and atrophy of his Bracing Muscles of the left hip. After we treated his back, we sent him to physical therapy to strengthen the Bracing Muscles of the hip and to improve his breathing. He came back to see us after a few weeks of physical therapy to tell us that he hated physical therapy. He said that the exercises were too easy. He didn't sweat, he didn't feel sore the next day, and an 80-year-old lady there was doing the same exercises as him. I explained to him that he was like a fifty-foot-tall tree that gets blown over in a windstorm. The trunk is huge, the tree is enormous, but the roots are shallow and the tree cannot support itself while smaller trees may do fine in the same storm. He scoffed at me and agreed to continue physical therapy. I didn't see him for over a year until he brought his wife in for a consultation on her pain. He told me that he trains many people on deadlifts and that "everyone in my gym does the old lady exercises!" He taught his students the exercises because "you can't build a stable second story on the house with a bad foundation."

When your Bracing Muscles are weak, and the String Muscles that compensate for them are strong, you can keep yourself out of pain—for a while. The problem comes when you get injured. It is like walking on a tightrope six feet off the ground. As long as you stay up there, everything is good. But getting back up on that rope is difficult if you fall off. When your Bracing Muscles are weak, you are breath-holding, and you lack flexibility and mobility. You are moving that tightrope higher and higher. Getting back on is hard once you fall off due to an injury. When you correct these issues, you are lowering that rope closer and closer to the ground. You may get injured and have problems, but you will find getting back in the game much easier.

EGO MUSCLES

The ego is your enemy when it comes to doing these deceptively simple exercises. Like the athlete mentioned above, patients anxious to recover quickly often want to pump iron. They want to get in, work out hard, and fix the problem. They want to show people how much weight they can lift. They want to go to the gym and look good. They want to look in the mirror and flex their muscles, which are getting bigger and bigger. Many are convinced that they know how to strengthen muscles, as they have worked out all their lives.

The fact is, they probably do know how to strengthen their muscles—Action Muscles. But Bracing Muscles, as you now know, are different. If you have worked out all of your life, you know how it feels to work out Action Muscles. But Tune Me doesn't feel anything like this—there is no muscle to flex, nothing to show off, and nothing to make you look better in the mirror. What does change is that you will get better. You will feel better, have less pain, and be more mobile.

Unfortunately, many people focus on their ego muscles instead of embracing Tune Me. That's because it is difficult to do Tune Me for months before you feel any gains. Also, the exercises are hard to get a handle on. It is far more difficult to focus on muscles that keep you from moving rather than moving Action Muscles. It becomes harder still when your ego muscles are fighting you every step of the way. You need to let go and trust in the process.

ZONE 2 TRAINING

Recently, we've seen a rise in a type of training known as "Zone 2," and it makes for a good comparison to strengthening Bracing Muscles. In Zone 2 training, the person exercising tries to keep their heart rate between 60 and 70% of their maximal heart rate. In this zone, 65% of calories burned come from fat; above this range, calories draw more from protein and other sources.[17] As such, Zone 2 training is proving to be very beneficial for fat loss. And yet, many people struggle to find the sweet spot—they can't walk fast enough to reach the target heart rate, and then they go above the target range when they break into a slow jog. A heart rate monitor is essential, as it is difficult for many to know if they are in the zone without this feedback. When they finish with the 30-minute workout the literature suggests, most people feel like they did not get a great workout and often plan a different workout for later.

Bracing Muscle strengthening presents a similar Goldilocks dilemma. Here, the physical therapist acts as the heart rate monitor. They can help you find that perfect exercise where you are both contracting the correct muscle (not too easy) and not compensating with String Muscles (not too hard). When finished, it will not have felt like a great workout. You can do a "workout" later, but don't let your ego push you to drop these exercises.

ASYMMETRY

The other problem with strengthening these muscles is asymmetry in strength between sides of the body. Most people are stronger on one side than the other. They have one leg stronger than the other and one arm stronger than the other. This can cause complications when it comes to Tune Me.

Imagine this scenario: You are a runner who regularly does 5K races. You have no pain at all. You run a few miles a day several times per week. Three to five times per year, you run a 5K race, and you do fine. Then, one day, a friend suggests you do a full marathon. You do your research and realize that you will have to train for this race. You formulate a plan to slowly increase your miles over the next several months. The first month goes great; you incrementally increase your mileage every week, and you are feeling good. You like the challenge and the community. You get heavily into the sport and make lots of friends. You visit online forums and read about carbohydrate loading and mile pacing. You pick out a marathon sticker to put on your car and look down on people in the fast food drive-thru. It is all so exhilarating.

Marathon preparation involves weekday training and a weekend "long run." Most marathons are on a Saturday, so you get yourself prepared by doing progressively longer runs each preceding Saturday as you get closer to the marathon.

Often, patients will see me as a sports medicine doctor after the eighteen-mile run, or even the thirteen-mile run. They'll say that they were doing just fine, but then they had their long run, and "something happened." They are now in pain.

Guess what? Nothing actually happened to you or those other runners. What happened was that you each hit a point at which you exposed your hidden weaknesses.

This is where asymmetry comes into play. Most people are stronger on one side than the other. This is not necessarily a problem, but it can be once you reach the point of exertion that exposes this weakness. The weakness on one side may not have been exposed at five miles or even ten miles, but then you get to the thirteenth mile or so, and the fatigue eventually starts to set in. The muscles in your left foot, right leg, or buttocks are worn out. The strong foot, leg, or buttocks are fine and can keep going, but the weaker side hits a wall and cannot keep up. The problem of weakness on one side was always there, but it wasn't exposed until you hit a certain point of fatigue. Past that point, and "suddenly," the pain and limping start.

The same goes for back pain, except instead of escalating your workout to the point where asymmetry is exposed, you get injured, and the weakness that develops exposes the asymmetry. The injury starts the downward spiral of pain causing weakness, which causes more pain, which causes more weakness, and on and on until it eventually exposes asymmetry in your Bracing Muscles' ability to stabilize. This becomes important when isolating Bracing Muscles during the first part of Tune Me. You have to be aware of any asymmetry in your Bracing Muscles so that you can devise a program to correct it.

FRETTING

As you get better at bracing exercises, think of it the way a musician would play their instrument: perfectly and effortlessly. They can do this because of the tremendous time they have spent practicing finger placement. If you examine the fingertips of the fretting hand of an accomplished guitar player, you will find very small calluses. The calluses are small because the guitarist places their fingers on the strings in the same way every time, and they know the various chords so well that they could find them in their sleep. They finger these chords perfectly; fingering them close to perfectly does not produce the exact sound they want, so they work hard at attaining perfection.

You should put the same commitment into your exercises. We want you to play your Body Guitar well. That means getting these exercises perfect and doing them until they are second nature. You are going to be doing them for a long time. Remember that with endurance muscles, you need to build blood flow to these muscles, which takes months.

We often see patients return six months after first treating them. Sometimes, the return visit is due to injury, but much more often, their follow-up is due to one of two causes. In the first, the patient finishes their 4–6 weeks of physical therapy, then quits doing their Bracing exercises altogether so they can get back to "normal" exercises. As mentioned previously, normal exercises are not enough, as you have not built up enough endurance to make it through the day. You will begin to compensate without even knowing you are compensating. It all quickly falls apart, and I see the patient back with the same problem.

I've personally fallen prey to this very pattern. I injured my right shoulder playing college football over 30 years ago. One day at practice, we were doing route running in shorts and helmets, and one of my teammates thought it would be funny to try to run through me when I wasn't expecting it. My right shoulder hurt, but it wasn't too bad. Over the next ten years, I would get tightness on the top of my shoulder and into my right neck. I was working at a clinic with Dr. Jim Andrews in Birmingham, Alabama, and he said, "Wheeler, your scapula is not sitting right; go see our physical therapist." I learned some exercises, I got them perfect, and the pain went away until six months later, when it came back. I returned to the exercises, and the pain went away for six months. I went through this cycle three times until I finally committed to building the necessary endurance strength.

The second six-month failure is the patient who does physical therapy and learns their exercises perfectly. They continue to do all these exercises faithfully, even increasing repetitions and time spent doing them. This patient then returns at six months with a recurrence of pain. The issue is that the patient has become so efficient and good at isolating the Bracing Muscle that they utterly fatigue the very muscle they need to use all day to stabilize and, instead, end up compensating for much of the day. So, our "perfect" patient ends up coming back with not only pain but also frustration. I have to explain that while we have to build strength initially, we reach enough strength to have an increased tone after just a couple of months. Then, by appropriately using this tone, we build the muscle further with our posture and walking. It sounds like I'm contradicting everything I have stated about endurance strength, doesn't it? What I would like to do is define a subtle difference.

When someone strengthens a weak Bracing Muscle, they need both initial strengthening to build tone and to activate this newly re-strengthened muscle so they can use it all day. Everyone starts from a different place of strength, so you cannot uniformly say how long it takes for a person to reach the point where muscles begin to have tone. Someone who has atrophy of the muscles, as we saw in the MRI of the previous chapter, will take a very long time. For the first 8–12 weeks after an injection, the steroid reduces the inflammation of the joint, but after this time, the lack of stability brought on by the fatigue leads to a return of joint or disc pain. Therefore, this very weak patient will probably require a repeat injection in 8–12 weeks to get a longer period to strengthen in the pain-free time zone. Maybe even a third injection. But eventually, in all patients, we will reach that point where tone is attained. You then don't necessarily get more tone by continuing to work out these small muscles. The continued workout can fatigue them and cause compensation. Instead, getting the body in the right posture and following the correct cues leads to all-day use of these muscles, increasing strength. But you can't just hope they will fire all day because they won't. The brain has developed new patterns of motion and, left without proper activation, will continue to compensate unless instructed not to, even when the Bracing Muscles are stronger. So, our patients do strengthening, and the brain still overuses the old compensating String Muscles. To overcome this, we have to activate the appropriate muscles each morning without fatiguing them.

Each morning, after stretching, I will do a right scapula strengthening exercise while brushing my teeth and a right gluteus exercise while making my coffee. Each takes me about a minute; I know how to do them perfectly, and I think of it as tuning my instrument before playing it all day. I may also do several other exercises, but over the years, I have found that I must do these two exercises, or I will find a way to compensate. Even after not having pain for years, I will compensate and fall into a bad pattern of motion. These exercises are unique to me, and every patient must find their patterns of motion and areas of weakness that are unique to them. We find this by investing in physical therapy. Not just going to physical therapy but entrenching yourself in therapy and learning how to do the exercises, how you compensate, and how you fall back into old patterns of motion.[18] I then invest in the Wheeler Walking Method you will find in the appendix as often as I can. That has proven to be a way for me to continue to strengthen my muscles over the long haul.

You especially need to be sure you are not breath-holding while doing your physical therapy exercises. For years, physical therapists have created breath-holders by allowing breath-holding during the exercises. The problem is that when you breath-hold, you are inhibiting the Bracing Muscles. Therefore, if you are breath-holding when doing exercises to build strength and endurance to the Bracing Muscles of the spine and hip, the only things you are strengthening are the String Muscles.

This requires a monumental shift in physical therapy practices, and in back pain patient's expectations of the physical therapist. In the first edition of this book, I discussed how patients were to build enough endurance in the Bracing Muscles so that they could contract all day. I suggested that they should contract their abdominal muscles and hold that contraction for much of the day. Those of us in the medical establishment who taught this were actually creating breath-holders. Instead, we have to stop breath-holding, strengthen the correct muscles to the point where we have increased the tone of those spring-like muscles. Then, the increased tone stabilizes us throughout the day without contraction or breath-holding.

> Appropriate muscle exercises for Bracing Muscles of the spine and of the hip. *(Placing the fingers on the guitar in exactly the right place)*

> Breathe with the stomach and not the chest, relax the spine and buttocks. *(Down-down-up—Up-down-up)*

Build a rhythm, and learn to play your instrument. Eventually, the unconscious orchestra of stability begins to return with appropriate breath-holding, Bracing Muscle tone, and String Muscle contraction when necessary.

You cannot play a guitar with one hand. You have to learn the finger placement and the strumming together. When you practice strengthening and abdominal breathing together, the Bracing Muscles of the spine, lower back, neck, hip, and feet get a better workout, and we are on the path to tuning our Body Guitar.

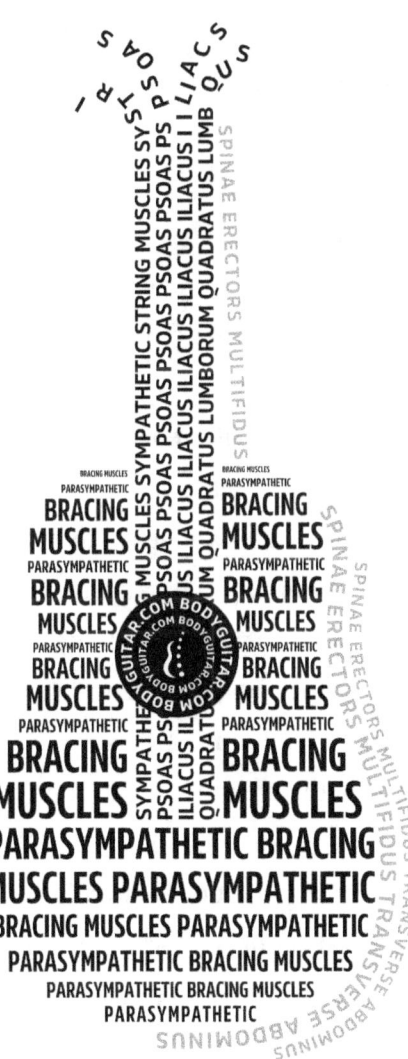

You need both to make the music you want. So, learn your exercises and proper breathing, and start doing both. You need strength to build tone. You need tone to get endurance. You need endurance to get better. The fretting hand exercises strengthen you while the strumming hand exercises limit inhibition, building tone. Commit to learning and being obsessed with both in the long term, because that is what it's going to take.

5. Tune Me: Feedback

We all need feedback. Every garage band thinks that they are the next Nirvana until they get constructive feedback from someone listening to their music. In the case of back pain, we have to look hard for feedback that is reliable. These muscles aren't getting bigger. We are doing great with the exercises, but don't feel any better. It can be very frustrating. The feedback I am going to describe to you is both encouraging to you on your journey and part of the final destination. It's encouraging because you now will have something that you can measure to keep you from getting frustrated.

The first feedback is posture. Everyone wants good posture; however, few people actually know what good posture looks like. When you ask someone to adopt good posture, they sit up taller and straighter. This is necessary to good posture, but good posture is so much more. Sitting up straight is a habit you can learn and a habit I want for you, but sitting up straight is nowhere near all that you need.

Let's now look at what good, healthy posture looks like. There are five key areas of good posture that can affect lower back pain:

- Stand/sit up straight
- Relax buttocks
- Normal arch to lower back
- Shoulders down and back
- Head over shoulders

After achieving these positions, there is one feedback that has to occur. If posture is a feedback, this is the feedback to the feedback. Stand up, holding the book; if you can't at this moment, come back to this page. As you stand, assume what you would consider good posture without doing any of the above cues. We will get to them. With your good military stance, are you on your heels or mid-foot? If you are on your heels, relax your butt and soften your knees. Are you on your heels or mid-foot? If you are on your heels, relax the arch of your back and breathe through your stomach. Are you on your heels or mid-foot? Now, try to get your head back over your shoulders. Are you on your heels or mid-foot? If you are on your heels, then instead of having the mobility to get your head in the right place, you have just arched your thoracic spine. Now, try dropping your shoulders down and back. Are you on your heels or mid-foot? If you are on your heels, you have gone too far back. Standing position is a great feedback when it comes to posture. We should be on our mid-foot or the arches of our feet for all positions. This means we have to diaphragmatically breathe, relax both buttocks and spine, and recognize where our weight is centered.

Learning to sit or stand up straight is a habit. Most people can learn this habit in a month or two. Posture is a test of the tone we have built back into our Bracing Muscles and a measure of our sympathetic tone.[19] As we strengthen the Bracing Muscles, we regain the spring-like tone in these muscles to hold us in position throughout the day. When we assume good posture, we are both strengthening these muscles and assessing their tone. We also are practicing our diaphragmatic breathing. If we are breath-holding, we will be on our heels. If our tone is not great, we will end up breath-holding and, thus, on our heels. If we arch our back to achieve our desired posture, we will be on our heels. These simple tests provide great feedback of both strumming hand and fretting hand.

Some hypermobile patients have adapted by locking their knees, pushing their pelvis forward, and overarching through their back. This is also not acceptable and has to be worked out through extensive work. There are actually many odd postures that we adopt throughout our lives, and a therapy professional is the best option to correct what is wrong, and begin to get on the right path.

During the feedback portion of Tune Me, your posture doesn't have to be perfect. In fact, it can't be. It has to flow with your day and adjust to every movement. Sitting at your desk, walking to meetings, climbing stairs, sitting at ballgames: through all of it, you work on this posture in many varied ways and positions. Eventually, you get to the point where it happens unconsciously. You use the correct muscles to stabilize yourself at all times because it feels right. You don't have to think about it; it is an extension of you.

FLEXIBILITY

To get into good posture, we have to have flexibility in certain muscles. Most of these muscles are also String Muscles. If these muscles are compensating, then the posture position is compromised.

Going from top to bottom, we can organize area by area. If the back of the neck is tight and the deep muscles of the neck are weak, then getting the head in the correct position without arching through the thoracic spine is difficult.

If the pec minor muscles are tight, then the scapula base is unstable, and getting the shoulders in the right spot is nearly impossible.

If the Bracing Muscles of the spine and hip are weak, then the hip flexors and hamstrings are tight, and we will resort to clenched butt muscles and breath-holding.

If the soleus and small muscles of the foot are weak, the feet are not in a great position to stabilize, and the feedback could be compromised.

Our flexibility feedback then becomes: the back of the neck, the pec minor, the hip flexors, the hamstrings, and the calf. Each of these should be flexible. As hyperflexible people are unable to use muscle tightness as feedback, posture and awareness of appropriate muscle weakness become even more important.

You will fail if you attempt to lengthen and increase flexibility in these String Muscles while your Bracing Muscles are weak.[20] You will stretch daily while making little gains. Then, if you take a day or two off from stretching, your muscles will return to being just as tight as they were before you ever stretched. They have to shorten to do the job your Bracing Muscles are not doing. As you realize some strength and endurance in these Bracing Muscles, you can stretch the String Muscles. The stretch will be easier, and the flexibility will remain. Again, we can use this feedback to measure our improvement. When the flexibility improves, you can be certain that you are getting stronger. If your flexibility is still bad, your endurance strength is still inadequate.

JOINT MOBILITY

The third and last feedback is joint mobility. Joint mobility is much like flexibility, but I bring it up last, not because you have to do it after everything else is completed, but because it is difficult to restore joint mobility without endurance, strength, and flexibility. You can begin working on thoracic spine mobility and hip joint mobility whenever you want, and I recommend that you do so from the very beginning, but this will be late feedback in that it could take a long time to have lasting results.

The recovery process is cyclic and graduated. More strength, flexibility, endurance, and mobility will feed off each other. You will discover that more mobility will help you to gain more endurance, strength, and flexibility. That's the great thing about Tune Me and pain recovery. Just as all of your problems coalesced and caused more problems exponentially, so does recovery as it begins to snowball. As you fix one issue, others will benefit. That is the glory of your Body Guitar—it all fits together like a wonderful, beautiful, amazing puzzle.

6. Achieve Your 180 in 180

As you can see, all of this takes time. You aren't going to observe significant progress in the first few months outside of your increased flexibility and posture duration. I am always a little hesitant to tell people this, because I don't want to discourage them. My hope is that it does the opposite: that this knowledge keeps you from getting discouraged in those first months when you are working hard but seeing little tangible results. What you need to realize is that, if you are working the system, you are actually getting results, even if you

People with chronic back pain developed that pain, and any accompanying weakness and immobility, over the course of their lives. You aren't going to undo all of that damage in the course of a day.

can't yet see them.

People with chronic back pain developed that pain, and any accompanying weakness and immobility, over the course of their lives. You aren't going to undo all of that damage in the course of a day. But if you work the system, rest assured that you are headed in the right direction. It just takes time to get there. This is not measured in days or weeks—but in months. You will continue to see improvement over months if you continue to work the system. But you have to commit yourself for the long haul. If you are awake for sixteen hours but only have enough endurance strength to be stable for twelve of those hours, you are not fully improved. You may still experience pain every day just because of those final four hours of instability.

Patients need to put in a minimum of 180 days to start seeing a turnaround.[21] This is how long it takes for most people to build enough strength in the Bracing Muscles to see a real change in the physical manifestations of their pain. After that time, you may not be 100 percent back to normal (not every patient ever achieves that level of success) and you may not have fully resolved your pain, but you will now be on the path to recovery. You can achieve a complete 180-degree turn in 180 days.

Please note: This 180-degree turn doesn't mean that you are back to where you started—it's a turn. It means you have reversed course and are now on the road to recovery. I hope that doesn't dispirit you. This is an ongoing, lifelong process. To return to the weight-loss metaphor I used earlier, sustained weight loss is never achieved by diet plans. Real, sustainable weight loss is only ever achieved by changing one's lifestyle. Likewise, Tune Me is not a rigorous 180-day workout meant to fix your back and allow you to return to your old ways; this is a new operating system for your body, one that must be attended to, updated, and maintained. You can't just "install" it and forget it.

I say that you will achieve your 180 in 180 in order to stress that this is not a passive process. Success means remaining dedicated to doing the exercises you learned with your physical therapist, maintaining good posture, abdominal breathing, and staying in contact with your doctor and physical therapist to make sure that progress is being made.

You can't just expect to go to physical therapy and have them fix you. They can help teach you how to play your Body Guitar, but only you can take what you learned home with you and put in the work. Your therapist can be like a music instructor, teaching you the scales and chords of your Body Guitar, but only you can take those lessons home and really utilize them. Achieving your 180 in 180 is about you taking the information and exercises that you learned in rehab over 4–6 weeks and incorporating them into many parts of your life.

When you see a new guitarist hold their guitar, it almost looks painful. Their wrists are bent uncomfortably, and they look like they are fighting the instrument. After six months, the guitarist and their instrument can produce some wonderful music—and, after several years, the guitar and the player look like they were made for each other. The guitar now appears to be an extension of the player. I want this for you. With six months of hard work, you should be able to accomplish good music. After several years, I want your body to be a physical extension of your soul.

So, give yourself those 180 days before you start making judgments about whether your treatment is working. There is no other way. If you give up before 180 days, you will never see results. You need that long to start turning the ship around—but you can get there.

One of the most important milestones of this journey will be reaching a point where you have gained enough endurance in the Bracing Muscles to maintain good posture for the entire waking day—a full sixteen hours. This can take a while to achieve, but you can get there. You will see steady progress, and while you may not see any changes in pain right away, you can track improvements in stability by using the feedback I described.

Beyond having our pain greatly reduced, our goal is to have great posture, breathing, flexibility, and joint mobility. After your Body Guitar is in tune, these feedback devices will begin to tell you if things are going wrong. If your posture, flexibility, breathing, or joint mobility worsens, it's an early warning signal that your Bracing Muscles are weakening.

LIVING TUNE ME

To briefly recap, Tune Me works like this: You start by seeing a doctor who will get you a proper diagnosis by performing a real hands-on physical exam. The doctor then treats your pain or recommends you to a specialist who can treat your pain. When you are able to settle into your spine without pain, you are able to switch from String Muscles to Bracing Muscles. These Bracing Muscles have atrophied if you have had pain for more than a couple of months, and you have lost postural muscle strength. You begin to work on abdominal breathing to decrease your sympathetic tone. Now, it is time to visit a physical therapist who will help you identify which Bracing Muscles are weak and then come up with an exercise program that isolates those muscles. Your physical therapist will help you learn about your body and teach you how to correctly play it by providing you with a set of exercises to work on. While doing this, you continue to work on other ways of decreasing your sympathetic tone by improving sleep and diet, along with increased exercise, and monitoring your sympathetic tone.

At this point, you will need to start tracking feedback to make sure you are progressing. From there, you will work toward achieving your 180 in 180 by spending 4–6 weeks strengthening, followed by at least six months working on a few of the exercises to increase strength while also practicing better posture and walking to increase endurance. This is the start to doing this for a lifetime. Meanwhile, you will also be working on flexibility and joint mobility throughout the process. Over time, you should see improvements in Bracing Muscle strength and endurance, as well as breathing, posture, mobility, and flexibility. Leading to a return of the seamless and beautiful interaction between Bracing Muscles, String Muscles, and breathing to create stability. We focus on all of these issues together with one ultimate goal in mind: addressing and fixing any instability in the back, which is what is causing your chronic back pain. None of this happens overnight, and improvements in stability, mobility, and muscle endurance do not happen in sequence. You have to focus on them all simultaneously because each problem causes a feedback loop. Begin strengthening exercises and improved posture as soon as you can in order to begin reversing any stability and immobility problems you have. As the Bracing Muscles get stronger, they will be better able to stabilize the body and improve flexibility, allowing for a more natural—and stable—posture.

Improving muscle endurance will drive your recovery. As your endurance increases, the Bracing Muscles will be able to stabilize the body for a little longer each day before the String Muscles, breath-holding, and poor posture take over for weak Bracing Muscles. As you continue to work out the Bracing Muscles, they will gain blood flow and endurance. After about six months of this, you should be at a point where you start to see real improvements in your chronic pain—improvements that can, if you keep living Tune Me, last a lifetime.

Imagine yourself as someone with excellent breathing, posture, flexibility, and joint mobility along with manageable back pain. Imagine yourself empowered in this process—empowered to control your destiny and realize the future you want for yourself. Tune

Me can get you there, if you work it. Tune Me will help you restring, re-strut and replay your Body Guitar and keep it in tune throughout your lifetime, so that you are free to play the pain-free life song that you want to play.

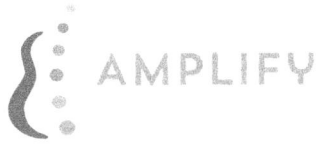 AMPLIFY

It has often been said that, to make discoveries, one must be ignorant. This opinion, mistaken in itself, nevertheless conceals a truth. It means that it is better to know nothing than to keep in mind fixed ideas based on theories whose confirmation we constantly seek, neglecting meanwhile everything that fails to agree with them..

—Dr. Claude Bernard, the father of modern medicine

Body Guitar and Tune Me have been used in my practice with my patients, people like you, over the last several years with great success. In my clinic, over 80% of patients who fully committed to Tune Me reported significant pain reduction within six months—a testament to its potential. This success was so great that it compelled me to write this book. I was also compelled by my patients, who told me that no one has ever explained their back in such a helpful way and given them an effective method to deal with their back pain. I was compelled by the residents I teach as they read through my unfinished manuscripts and pushed me to finish this book. I was compelled by an early editor who helped me organize my thoughts and told me that I had to finish this book because the world deserved to know this information.

I was compelled by the hopeless research that says that nothing works when it comes to treating chronic back pain. I was compelled by the insurance companies that wanted me to treat patients according to a failed and flawed treatment algorithm.

All of this compelled me to put this book out there now in order to share and amplify the message, even if it meant bypassing the more accepted routes of disseminating new medical knowledge. People are suffering, and we need a revolution right now. Everyone wants this and needs this: patients, doctors, researchers, everyone—even the insurers.

AMPLIFY THE REVOLUTION

When musicians want to crank up the volume, they turn to amplification as the answer. They plug in and turn up the volume. By using an amplifier, you can make your music heard far and wide.

This book opened with a discussion of a "revolution of one" that must happen in you. The revolution can't wait for the medical establishment to catch up. We all need to start a revolution in our own lives. The first step is you reclaiming your own life and living your personal uprising. This book is supposed to change your life, and allow you to play your life song—the song of your life that you were meant to play before back pain derailed you. By merely playing this life song, by living up to your potential, you will help to amplify this book. You will be its greatest testament.

But the revolution of one is only the first step. The second step is to join together and make our voices heard—we want to amplify each other. With each new convert, we get a little louder and a little harder to ignore. Your voice will join others in a great chorus. My hope is that when enough patients get on board, their doctors, physical therapists, and insurance companies will also get on board, and the movement will begin to build. Each of our voices will amplify one another and drive real change.

AMPLIFY THE MESSAGE TO PATIENTS

As a patient, you are the heart of this revolution. This book is your revolution—your liberation from back pain. By living Tune Me and understanding your Body Guitar, you can live a new life free from pain.

You can be active in this amplification process. Place demands on your physician. Place demands on your physical therapists. Ask your

The only way to tackle systemic illnesses like chronic back pain is for patients and healthcare providers to work together. I hope that this book changes the way doctors think.

doctor: "How will we address my Bracing Muscle weakness?" Show your PT this book and ask: "Can you teach me to isolate my muscles without breath-holding?" Hold them to better standards of care. The only way to tackle systemic illnesses like chronic back pain is for patients and healthcare providers to work together. I hope that this book changes the way doctors think. What I know is that, if patients everywhere come together and start demanding better care, they will get it.

I ask you now—join the movement. Inform your doctor. Inform your physical therapist. Evangelize not just to your healthcare providers, but also to other people. People who could benefit from Tune Me are everywhere. When, after six months of working Tune Me, you see a substantial breakthrough in your own health and pain levels, share that breakthrough with someone else. Post your 180-day progress online or tell a friend over coffee—just don't overpromise without guiding them to a professional. There are millions of people suffering, often silently, with chronic low back pain. They are desperate for answers and new solutions, just like you. Don't keep what you know from them. Get out there and spread the word. Tell them about this book, point them to the website www.BodyGuitar.com, and loan them your copy of this book.

You don't have to have back pain to be affected by Body Guitar and Tune Me. Once you know you have a Body Guitar and understand the principles of Tune Me, you have begun to know your body better. This knowledge will help you to keep your Body Guitar from ever falling out of tune if you are injured or develop poor posture. Everyone can benefit from this proactive prevention. The way you stand, the way you sit, and the way you move now can always improve and should always be monitored knowledgeably.

AMPLIFY THAT PREVENTION IS BETTER THAN TREATMENT

Everyone and every industry should focus on prevention because the lifestyle choices that lead to back pain are endemic to our society. We sit constantly—Americans average over 10 hours daily, according to the CDC—at work, at home in front of the TV, while we eat and read. We sit for the majority of the day, and all of this sitting changes our posture. This position may not cause back pain in and of itself, but it sets us up for chronic pain if we happen to get hurt.

Good preventative care for back pain needs to focus on reducing the amount of time we spend sitting. Stand-up desks are a good start. Screening tests throughout our lives that measure our posture or Bracing Muscle strength could become as common as screening for scoliosis or blood pressure. Posture checks at 5, 10 and 15 could catch deviations early. Flexibility, correct breathing, and posture could become more emphasized in grade school P.E. class as the Body Guitar concepts become more mainstream.

My three-year-old daughter had perfect posture. Her head was in a correct position, and her muscles and joints were flexible. As she is now 13, she does not have perfect posture. This begs the questions: Do these changes begin with school, as we "chain" kids to a chair for many hours a day? Does posture naturally change as kids grow and get bigger and stronger than their toddler Bracing Muscles can stabilize? Is it these things, plus others? We need to know. We need to stop allowing our kids to develop flawed posture. We allow them to have flawed posture, weak Bracing Muscles, and reduced mobility and flexibility, and then expect them to go on to be pain-free as adults. Is there an age where we need to work harder on posture that would make a huge difference? How about flexibility? When do we screen kids for compensatory Action Muscle use? Since we are a society that sits, we have become a society of back pain sufferers. The time has come to begin combating the effects of sitting from a young age and any other modern lifestyle choices that may be leading to back pain. We either have to sit less or work on getting our posture in a position that combats constant sitting. Whatever we do, we need to take action as a society.

People in blue-collar jobs must learn how to do their jobs while being stable. Many construction workers spend their lives with physically demanding jobs, and they come to see me dressed in suspenders because their buttocks have disappeared and they now have back pain. They have lost their gluteus muscles, and their backs are unstable. This is not from a lifetime of sitting, but a lifetime of minor injuries that leads to Bracing Muscle weakness. They are hurt and in pain, but they still have to get the job done any way they can. If they were taught how to deal with injuries, how to preserve their Bracing Muscles, not to breath-hold when they shouldn't, and how to use their posture to prolong their careers pain-free, we would be making radical changes in their career durations.

Pregnant women must be taught that they need to get their Bracing Muscle strength back after they deliver their child—and they need to do this before back pain kicks in. People with abdominal surgeries need the same rehab.

Anyone with an injury that requires surgery must be shown how to maintain their Bracing Muscle strength during the period of injury that causes them to remain inactive, so they don't lose that needed Bracing Muscle endurance. Sports injuries should be diagnosed with both the acute injury in mind plus the long-term strength issues. Sports injuries should be treated to prevent losing Bracing Muscle strength from the time of initial injury, so that they don't lose strength while healing from the initial injury.

Every break in activity due to injury or anything else must be thought of in two ways: treat the pain and then address long-term complications before they are problems. We already treat the short-term pain and injuries, but we are ignoring the long-term implications these problems present, such as Bracing Muscle weakness, that occur whenever we are not active. Understanding the relationship between sympathetic tone, inflammation, sleep, stress, and other factors needs to be addressed before we develop back pain.

AMPLIFY THE MESSAGE TO THE
INSURANCE INDUSTRY

The insurance industry wants different solutions to the problem of chronic back pain. They understand that what we are currently doing is not working—not for enough people—but they don't know what to do about it. Insurers are trying to find the most cost-effective way to cure patients while not continuing to treat the people who are "never" going to get better. They look to the pain societies to tell them which procedures and practices work, what should be the standard of care, and which medical practices are best for helping the most possible people.

After implementing these recommended practices, insurers review the numbers to make sure that they are working. Believe it or not, your insurance company wants you to be healthy, but they can't go bankrupt paying for procedures in a futile attempt to get you there. When they review the numbers showing how effective the treatments they pay for are, the numbers are not good when it comes to back pain treatment. So, it should be no surprise that they don't want to pay for ineffective treatments.

There has to be a cost-effective way to treat chronic back pain. Body Guitar and Tune Me are the way. Preventing one chronic case could save $50,000 in lifetime treatments verses $5,000 in proactive rehab—a no-brainer for insurers. The only real variables in Body Guitar are you, the patient, and your motivation to complete endurance strengthening—these things can affect the effectiveness of treatment. Despite the uncertainty created by these big variables, Tune Me works, and it is cost-effective. The insurance industry will change to a more cost-effective approach, if given one.

As Tune Me and Body Guitar are amplified, they will be adopted, and two things will happen: there will be an aggressive approach to the treatment of back pain and an aggressive approach to the prevention of back pain.

Insurers will make sure that back pain is treated aggressively because it is in their financial interest. It is the only cost-effective solution. Insurance companies will encourage multi-specialty approaches that direct care towards the periods of pain relief during which strengthening treatment occurs. They will encourage better posture, breathing, and Bracing Muscle physical therapists and trainers. They will incorporate other specialists who can provide temporary relief and long-term mobility and flexibility, which increase our ability to recover lost strength and endurance and, ultimately, stability.

Insurance companies will also begin to focus more on prevention when they realize how cost-effective it is to prevent back pain rather than to treat it—especially as patients demand it.

AMPLIFY THE MESSAGE TO THE MEDICAL COMMUNITY

My hope is that this book has illuminated a new path for the current treatment of back pain, inviting us to refine our approach together. So much must change. The diagnosis and treatment of back pain must change. The treatment algorithm must be ditched, while the understanding that one thing causes another must be embraced. Physicians must work towards making better and more accurate diagnoses. The focus of treatment must be on the rapid improvement of pain with a quick transition into strengthening. Our use of and understanding of MRI changes must become more in line with what we find on the physical exam. Our understanding of the kinetic chain must become better. One of the most neglected topics in medical school is the musculoskeletal exam—this, too, must change. Physicians must know what they are expecting from good physical therapists and demand it. They must know how to use a massage therapist and others, in a combined effort to get patients back to strengthening. Diagnostic skills must improve.

Physical therapists must learn to send people who are still hurting back to physicians, rather than spending their valuable time on modalities and not treating their weaknesses. Physical therapists must become experts on muscle isolation and kinetic chain abnormalities. They must be able to teach people how to fire the correct muscle without breath-holding, how to identify sympathetic and parasympathetic balance, how to overcome the nervous system and fear of motion, and how to motivate patient compliance over the long term. They must learn to work with professionals who can help with pain relief, muscle fascia breakdown, flexibility, and joint mobility in an effort to build a pain-free window in which patients can work on improving stability.

Patients should leave physical therapy with a complete and thorough understanding of posture, breathing, and exercises that they can use for a lifetime without having to return to physical therapy.

Trainers must become versed in a new way of using exercises to identify Bracing Muscle weakness. Bracing Muscle strength should be included in not only every workout routine, but also in every exercise. Joint mobility and flexibility should not be just for people with low back pain, but for everyone. Physical therapists are a necessity for all people with profound Bracing Muscle weakness and pain who are overusing sympathetic String Muscles. Trainers are for people without pain, but these trainers must be able to recognize when to send someone to a physical therapist. They must recognize when someone is overusing their String Muscles and how to get them to quit. If they cannot, they need to learn to work with a physical therapist.

Exercise programs for people who have been inactive for an extended period of time should start with a 180-day plan for building stability, flexibility, joint mobility, and cardiovascular health while slowly adding in more Action Muscle work to prevent people from getting hurt. The number of people who start working out at a gym only to get hurt is way too high. These people are trying to build a second story on their "house" when their foundation is cracked. Let's start them on the right path by getting the "foundation" of their Bracing Muscles some endurance before trying to build up the Action Muscles. By doing this, more trainers' clients will stay healthy and return for more workouts. The effect on their clients will be more than just getting in shape.

The medical community is vast and has many participants. It will be difficult to get them to all come together, but it is what must be done—and patients amplifying their demands can help us unite.

AMPLIFY THE NEED FOR RESEARCH

The publication of *UPRISE* is only the beginning. I fully admit that I don't have all of the answers. I have a new set of concepts and theories with some clear value, but we need more discoveries—an explosion of discoveries. I don't want to "own" these concepts and keep them to myself. If I did, I would not have published this book. What I want is for these ideas to go out into the world and be amplified by other doctors, proactive patients, researchers, and all of the medical community. I want everyone to advance the treatment of this problem together.

Until the research begins to rally around this concept, it will remain a "crazy" idea. Tune Me is too effective for it to remain a fringe practice. It needs to go mainstream, but for that to happen, statistics and studies will have to prove the effectiveness and results that I see in my own practice. I challenge the academic world to take this on, not as a confrontation, but as a collaboration.

- Studies that have shown no long-term benefit of spinal

procedures will have to be repeated, this time taking into account the time that the procedure gives the patient to get Bracing Muscle strength and whether the patient has complied with rehab. There are numerous incredible studies out there that were well-intentioned but imperfectly designed. They were asking the wrong questions and looking for the wrong outcomes.

Other studies needed include:

- Proving that facet pain leads to SI joint pain.
- Gait changes because of pain lead to more areas of pain.
- The physical exam is useful and essential when applied to low back pain.
- Steroids can provide pain relief long enough to get through rehab.
- Use of MRI in pain management and results.
- Long-term results of radiofrequency ablation of facet joints.
- Along with a host of other studies that can be gleaned from this book.

I also propose a theory to propel research forward.

The Body Guitar Theory:

1. Bracing Muscles are high-tone endurance muscles

that provide static stability and posture. These muscles provide parasympathetic stability and balance with sympathetic String Muscles to create complex muscular balance to the spine and other areas of the body.

2. When these muscles weaken, the body compensates to recreate stability, and these compensations prevent adults from regaining Bracing Muscle strength.

3. In the lumbar spine and hip, where stability is of utmost importance, breath holding and String Muscles become the dominant mode of stability when back pain persists.

4. Increased sympathetic tone and String Muscles of the lumbar spine cause inhibition of Bracing Muscles, leading to increased weakness and a cycle of back and/or hip pain and weakness.

5. To regain Bracing Muscle strength, strengthening must involve relaxation of String Muscles to allow full and unopposed contraction of the Bracing Muscles.

Now that the underlying cause of chronic back pain has been put into a theory, let's get to work on testing it so that we can prove, once and for all, what causes back pain and what effectively treats it.

This is a challenge to all researchers, but not a confrontational challenge. I want us to come together and do this. The revolution beckons you.

WHAT'S NEXT?

Tune Me isn't just about lower back pain, but about the way we use our bodies and our relationship with our own health. You can boil everything down to one takeaway point: chronic back pain is only a symptom of a larger problem. Back pain is caused by all kinds of problems, but what drives recurrent, chronic back pain is weakness in the Bracing Muscles (especially those of the lumbar spine and hip area) that cause instability in the back.

The reason people don't get better is because, while Bracing Muscle weakness sets in quickly (often in less than a month), it takes a solid six months of exercises and better posture to regain tone and endurance. And none of this can happen if we continue to compensate with increased sympathetic tone. Most patients aren't able to ever get that lost strength back because they think strengthening the Bracing Muscles is about strength training—and it's not; it's about circulation training. It's about restoring blood flow and circulation to the Bracing Muscles. The only way to do this is to make Tune Me your body's new operating system. You have to learn to not just adopt the system, but really live it in all ways. Only this will permanently address the immobility, muscle weakness, instability, and, yes, *also the chronic back pain* that has been keeping your body out of tune and disrupting the music of your life.

LET THE CONVERSATION CONTINUE

This book is only the start of an ongoing dialogue with the greater medical community. That community includes patients, too. We want to change how medical academia, insurers, patients, doctors, and others within the healthcare community come together to address the world's leading cause of disability: chronic back pain.

To do so, we must uproot fifty years of established medicine in order to bring this ideology to fruition. This will be a process that will take a long time to unfold as the revolution grows and new research is undertaken. We will carry this knowledge far and wide. Also, we will improve upon the concepts of this book over time, as Tune Me is expanded and refined in light of new research and medical advances.

The conversation initiated by this book is only the beginning. You are invited to join me at www.BodyGuitar.com, where the conversation about how to ensure your personal UPRISE will continue.

REVOLUTION FROM BACK PAIN

Thank you for reading with an open mind. I hope this book helps you to live better today, as well as every day to come. This is, after all, a book about hope and healing. This book is your UPRISE—your liberation from back pain. By living Tune Me and understanding your Body Guitar, you can live a new life free from pain.

Live well, get better, and learn to play your life song. But keep coming back to partake in the conversation, because when it comes to back pain, we now know that hope has a new name.

Body Guitar®.

> **Live well, get better, and learn to play your life song.**

POSTURE

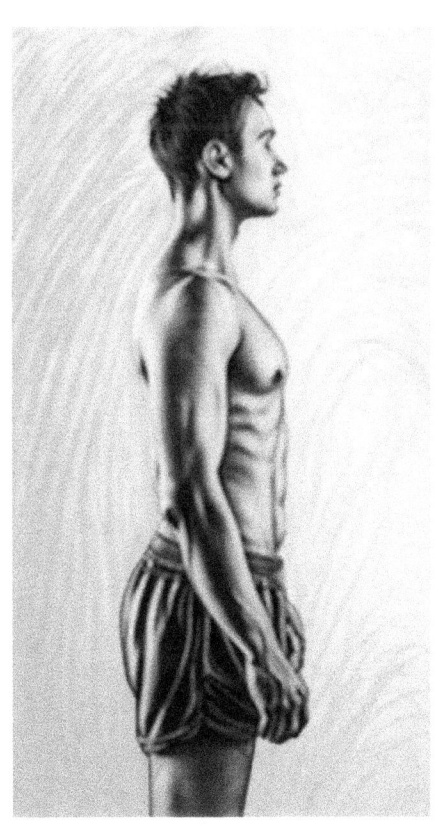

1. EARS APPROXIMATELY OVER SHOULDERS

2. NORMAL RELAXED CURVE IN THE LOWER BACK

3. STERNUM STRAIGHT UP AND DOWN

4. WEIGHT EVENLY DISTRIBUTED ON MID FOOT, NOT ON HEELS

5. BUTTOCKS RELAXED

6. KNEES RELAXED

EXERCISE SAMPLES

These examples are merely suggestions intended to be discussed with your physical therapist. They are not suitable for everyone and should not be used to replace professional therapy.

In each exercise, maintain proper posture and abdominal breathing to ensure that you are not relying on string muscles to compensate. If you allow string muscles to dominate, then the bracing muscles will not engage correctly.

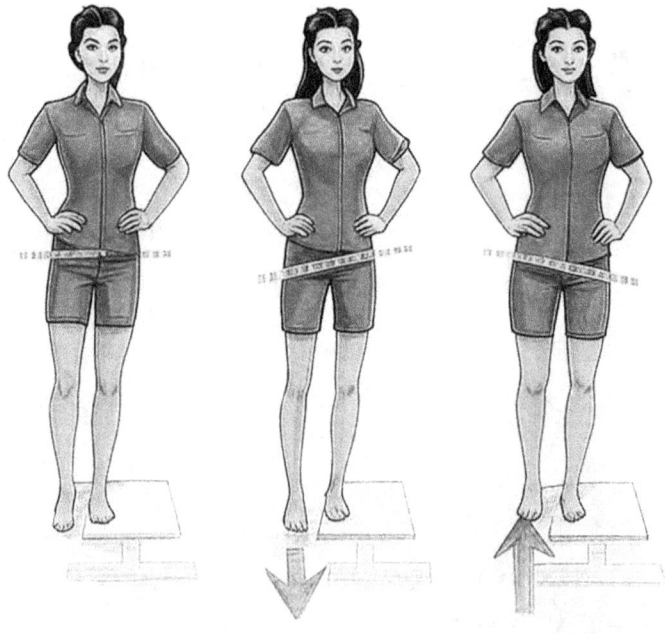

Hip Hike: This exercise targets the bracing muscles of the hip on the side that is on the step, not the moving side (the side that is providing stability to the movement). Keep both knees straight. Breathe through your nose to activate abdominal breathing. Relax your buttocks. This exercise primarily strengthens the gluteus medius and minimus muscles, which, raise your hip in preparation of the leg swinging through during walking. Start with 10 reps per leg per day and only progress to a maximum of 25.

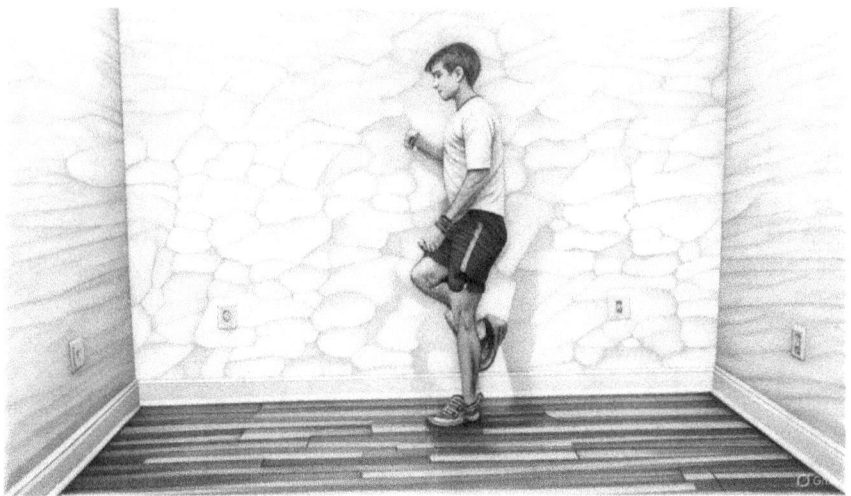

Wall Press: Press your knee into the wall to activate the external rotator on the side that is not pressing into the wall. Breathe with your diaphragm. You cannot activate the external rotator if the string muscles are pulling on the hip. Start with 10 seconds and 2 reps, advancing slowly. This is not a long-term exercise. It is designed to strengthen muscles enough to support the walking program below.

Bird Dog: This is one of McGill's "Big Three" exercises, but with one caveat. You must use abdominal breathing with this exercise. The multifidus and string muscles cannot be forcefully activated simultaneously. Maintain a normal arch in your back while doing this exercise and feel the vertebrae "settle in" to each other as you perform the exercise. If you are forcing this to happen, you are likely performing the exercise incorrectly. Extend the opposite arm and leg.

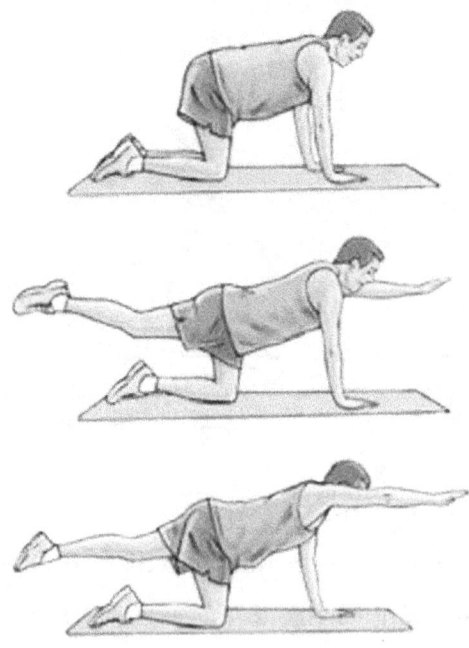

In each of these exercises, you may compensate as you fatigue (or even before then). If you do not recognize your compensations, you will not strengthen correctly. Empower yourself by seeking professional guidance.

Wheeler Walking Method: I recently traveled with my family to visit my daughter, Ellie, who was studying in London. While there, I did a lot of walking. Walked extensively—about 13 miles a day. We visited Buckingham Palace, Big Ben, Tower Bridge, Westminster Cathedral, along with numerous pubs and so many other sites. As I walked, I reflected on the principles outlined in this book. I also thought about how many of my patients were willing to do physical therapy, but with the goal of being more active.

While walking through London with my wife, I observed her very relaxed gait and excellent posture. As a seasoned distance runner, her gait reflected a parasympathetic dominated distance-running attitude. In contrast, as a former sprinter, my gait was much more front-side dominant: arms and feet more forward, stomach tight, with a sympathetic sprinting attitude. Over time, I began to imitate her walk. This adjustment activated my bracing muscles, stretched my hip flexors, reduced my sympathetic tone and improved my breathing and posture all through thoughtful walking. I realized that my patients could learn this type of walking to achieve several goals: exercise, strengthening, posture, breathing, and preparation for their own travels.

There is much to learn in this walking style, so take one step at a time and don't move on to the next step until you have mastered the previous one. Consider completing ten 20 minute walks before advancing.

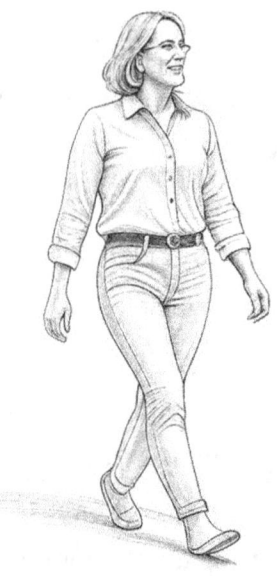

Step 1: Begin by standing with the posture we described in chapter 6 and above. Stand tall, relax your buttocks, breathe through your nose to relax your diaphragm, keep your knees soft without bending them, and settle into your mid foot and lower back. Ensure that your weight is not on your heels.

As you begin to walk, stay relaxed. Continue settling into your mid-foot and spine. Focus on posture, breathing and landing on your mid foot. Goals: Posture, breathing, mid-foot landing.

Step 2: After mastering step 1 through your repeated walks, focus on activating the bracing muscle of the hip. You cannot activate these muscles if you are breath-holding (chest breathing), as the string muscles will dominate. To engage the hip muscles, roll over your great toe (the big toe). As illustrated above, the leg that is behind her is firing her gluteus medius and minimus as the hip prepares to lift to allow the leg to swing through. The leg that is in front of her is firing her external rotator to keep her knee from collapsing inward. Each step alternates between the external rotator (lower butt) and gluteus medius/minimus (upper butt). Place your thumb on your upper butt and fingers on your lower butt to feel each of them contracting sequentially as you walk, provided you are in parasympathetic mode. Also, work on head posture by aligning your ears over your shoulders. The temptation that occurs as you continue walking and advancing in this protocol is to push your pelvis forward and lean back further. This is a fatal mistake in that it ruins much of what we are trying to accomplish. If this happens, it may be because the tone in your core muscles are weak. The compensation of this position is often to draw your stomach in. This is also a mistake as it leads to breath-holding and increased sympathetic tone. The solution is to keep yourself from doing either of the above flaws and to work on core strength when you are not walking to build thoughtless tone.

Goals: Same as Step 1, plus rolling over the great toe to activate the bracing muscles of the hip and head posture.

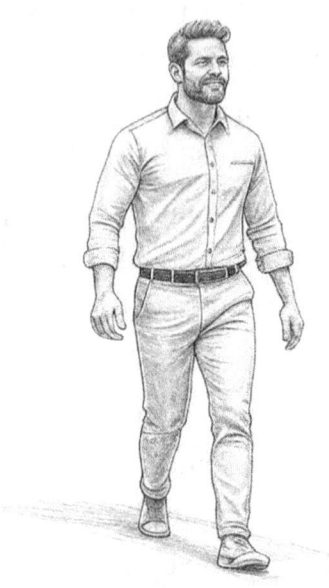

Step 3: This step is for long walks and is challenging if you are still consciously focusing on Steps 1 and 2. By lengthening your arm swing backward while keeping the forward swing normal, you also lengthen your steps behind you. By lengthening your steps behind you, we begin to stretch your hip flexors. This should be a natural, slightly exaggerated backward arm swing and should not feel uncomfortable. This hip flexor stretch is important as it counteracts a whole day of hip flexor tightness. Many patients have reported how this step took them from wanting to get their walk in daily to needing to get their daily walk. Don't jump ahead to this. Each step has to be completed, realizing that we go from unconsciously doing things wrong, to consciously doing things wrong, to consciously do-

ing things right, to unconsciously doing things right. Only when we get to this unconsciously right should we move on to the next step.

Goals: Same as Steps 1 and 2, plus stretch of hip flexors (psoas, iliacus)

Step 4: Now we need to get a little shoulder movement. This shoulder movement should be opposite to the hip rotation. (Right shoulder forward as left hip is back, and vice versa) This is also a normal walking motion, but people with back pain or who are older stop doing it. Watch a group of people walking and notice how many people have no shoulder movement. As you move your shoulders, you will begin to get much more multifidus activation. Be careful, as this can also irritate your facet joints, so start with one minute of shoulder rotation and advance very slowly. Also work more on posture as you are walking. Goals: Same as Steps 1–3, plus we are trying to get the shoulders moving to activate the multifidus.

With all these steps, we are activating our parasympathetic system and decreasing the sympathetic system. We are strengthening the gluteus and multifidus muscles. We are stretching your hip flexors and working on posture. Give us feedback on our website on this Wheeler Walking Method as it is forever a work in progress and I need feedback to make it better and better.

EMERGENCY TREATMENT

As you go through the Tune Me System, you will have some bad days. Sometimes this means that your original pain is back, and you need to see your doctor. But sometimes it just means that your string and bracing muscles are out of balance. One of them has been fatigued by your activity, and the other is screaming at you. We must begin to realize that there is a chronically out-of-balance state (this entire book is about this chronic state) and an acutely out-of-balance state. In the chronically state, you have major work to do. In the acute state, you have to stop the string muscle spasm so that the balance returns. This acute state is sometimes found in the person who doesn't have back pain and just over did it. But much more often it is found in the chronic back pain patient who is on the road to recovery, but just over did it. In these cases, I want to give you a plan to treat your acute pain so that you don't think that this is a return to the pain you had.

Step 1: You have to assume that the psoas is in spasm. In this case, getting the psoas to stop spasming will help. In this book, we mentioned numerous treatments for the psoas, and I would recommend using any of them: Chiropractic care, John Sarno's protocol, inversion table, etc. They are all listed, and perhaps more will come out. They are a great way to stop string muscle spasm. I also recommend that my patients learn how to release their own psoas. There are videos on YouTube, and I will put one on my website on how to effectively do this. Remember, your pushing on the psoas does not release it. But pushing on the psoas allows your brain to know that the psoas is tight so that you can consciously relax it. All of these psoas muscle treatments are acute-state muscle treatments. They are misused as chronic-state muscle treatments, so we must understand the difference.

Step 2: If this does not take care of the problem, then your gluteus muscles are fatigued and in spasm. Because they are not doing their job in stabilizing the hip, the string muscles are forced to take over. The spasm of the gluteus muscles is very common when someone with chronic back pain tries to get back to activity too early. I want my patients to increase activity, so developing gluteus muscle spasm and throwing the Body Guitar off balance is probably the sign of a good thing.

The way I ask my patients to treat this is with a lacrosse ball, but almost any ball will work. You roll the ball on the gluteal muscles until you find an area of pain. You increase the pressure, stay there until the muscle releases, and then move to find a new area. Again, I will put an explanation video on the website.

Step 3: We must work on decreasing sympathetic tone. Practice abdominal breathing. Go for a light, relaxing walk. Explore many other possible sympathetic tone remedies. Again, check the website, as we are building a back pain resource site.

If these don't help, and a few days of treatment aren't helping, contact your healthcare professional, as the chronic pain could be back. If the pain is severe, you may do that as the first step. I am trying to give you tools to manage your back pain on your own, but I am not asking you to use this book as a substitute for a health professional. Always use the advice given here as a supplement to advice from a qualified professional.

180 IN 180®

A 180 degree refocus in how you care for your back—requiring 180 days to unlearn what you think you know about low back pain— your BODY GUITAR—and to understand and begin relying upon the Tune Me operating system—to achieve Pain Liberation.

ACTION MUSCLE™

Movement muscles that appear throughout your body, one of two types of human muscle; Action Muscles trigger movement through-out your body, and are EITHER endurance muscles or ballistic muscles. You strengthen your Action Muscles by moving them. If your Bracing Muscles are not functioning properly, Action Muscles are called upon to compensate for weakness in your Bracing Muscles.

AMPLIFY

The fuller enjoyment of your life with those you care about and love as a result of understanding your BODY GUITAR, and the sharing of what you have learned to affect good health change.

BODY GUITAR™

The beautiful instrument that your body is, including your lumbar spine (low back) String Muscles and your Bracing Muscles—working together to create stability in an unstable area. Sympathetic large segment stability and parasympathetic small segment stability working much like an acoustic guitar to provide balance.

BRACING MUSCLE™

Stabilizing postural muscles in six different areas of your body, including your lumbar spine, your low back. Bracing Muscles are unique in many respects and are very important in developing coordination. When we hurt, these are the muscles that rapidly weaken and strengthening of these muscles determines our recovery from pain.

BRACING

Breath-holding to stabilize the spine when lifting something heavy. It is using diaphragm contraction to lock the String Muscles in place. Not related to Bracing Muscles except that both provide static stability.

BREATH-HOLDING

In this book, it is not technically holding your breath as you can still breathe with your chest. It is forceful contraction of the abdominal string muscles, thereby locking the diaphragm in place to create stability. Much like bracing, but bracing is additive onto normal stability. Breath-holding is only for fight-or-flight and when used all the time creates a spine imbalance.

CIRCULATION TRAINING™

A series of movements and exercises, performed regularly, that work to increase circulation—blood flow—to your Bracing Muscles; required for good health and quality of life as you age.

PAIN LIBERATION

The benefit your experience by understanding your BODY GUITAR and your use of Tune Me, creating your UPRISE.

PUMPING BLOOD

The result of Circulation Training, which increases regular blood flow to your Bracing Muscles so they will reflexively perform effectively for you.

SYMPATHETIC TONE

In the book it has to do with overuse of String Muscles. This overuse along with pain, leads to over expression of all of the components of "fight-or-flight" including increased cortisol production leading to sympathetic overload.

TUNE ME™

The OS or operating system for your BODY GUITAR. The Tune Me Method involves treating the pain, decreasing sympathetic tone, strengthening the Bracing Muscles, using appropriate feedback to monitor and putting the necessary time to effect a long-term change. It is an overall plan to use the information in this book to effect a lifelong back pain solution.

UPRISE

Your ability to move—to rise up and move in any direction—every day with little or no low back pain, which we label Pain Liberation; the outcome of your use of Tune Me.

● ● ●

* These terms are further defined at
http://bodyguitar.com/vernacular-glossary.html

Introduction

1   Foster, N. E. (2011). "Barriers and Progress in the Treatment of Low Back Pain." *BMC Medicine*, 9:108.

2   Maher, C., Underwood, M., & Buchbinder, R. (2017). "Non-specific Low Back Pain." *The Lancet*, 389(10070):736–747.

Chapter 1: Challenge

1   Husky, M. M., et al. (2018). "Chronic Back Pain and Its Association with Quality of Life in a Large French Population Survey." *Health and Quality of Life Outcomes*, 16:195.

2   Hartvigsen, J., Hancock, M. J., Kongsted, A., et al. (2018). "What Low Back Pain Is and Why We Need to Pay Attention." *The Lancet*, 391(10137):2356–2367.

3   Fatoye F, Gebrye T, Ryan CG, Useh U, Mbada C. Global and regional estimates of clinical and economic burden of low back pain in high-income countries: a systematic review and meta-analysis. *Front Public Health*. 2023 Jun 9;11:1098100. doi: 10.3389/fpubh.2023.1098100. PMID: 37383269; PMCID: PMC10298167.

4   Wu A, March L, Zheng X, et al. Global low back pain prevalence and years lived with disability from 1990 to 2017: estimates from the Global Burden of disease study 2017. *Ann Transl Med*. 20120;8(6):299

5   Shmagel, A., et al. (2019). "Chronic Back Pain in U.S. Adults: Prevalence and Impact on Everyday Activities." *Journal of Pain Research*, 12:1659–1666.

6   Lucas, J. W., et al. (2021). "Back, Lower Limb, and Upper Limb Pain Among

U.S. Adults, 2019." *NCHS Data Brief,* No. 415.

7   Urits, I., et al. (2019). "Low Back Pain, a Comprehensive Review: Pathophysiology, Diagnosis, and Treatment." *Current Pain and Headache Reports,* 23(3):23

8   Manchikanti, L., et al. (2021). "Lumbar Epidural Injections in the Treatment of Chronic Low Back Pain: A Systematic Review and Update." *Pain Physician,* 24:E645–E689

9   Is Creativity in Back Pain Research in Short Supply? Is Genius Extinct? *The Back Letter* 28(4):p 41, April 2013. | DOI: 10.1097/01.BACK.0000429083.32635.90

10   GBD 2021 Low Back Pain Collaborators. (2023). "Global, Regional, and National Burden of Low Back Pain, 1990–2020, Its Attributable Risk Factors, and Projections to 2050: A Systematic Analysis of the Global Burden of Disease Study 2021." *The Lancet Rheumatology,* 5(6):e316–e329. DOI: 10.1016/S2665-9913(23)00098-X

11   Hoy, D., et al. (2014). "The Global Burden of Low Back Pain: Estimates from the Global Burden of Disease 2010 Study." *Annals of the Rheumatic Diseases,* 73(6):968–974. DOI: 10.1136/annrheumdis-2013-204428

12   Maher, C., Underwood, M., & Buchbinder, R. (2017). "Non-specific Low Back Pain." *The Lancet,* 389(10070):736-747. DOI: 10.1016/S0140-6736(16)30970-9

13   Foster, N. E. (2011). "Barriers and Progress in the Treatment of Low Back Pain." *BMC Medicine,* 9:108. DOI: 10.1186/1741-7015-9-108

14   Buchbinder, R., et al. (2018). "Low Back Pain: A Call for Action." *The Lancet,* 391(10137):2384–2388. DOI: 10.1016/S0140-6736(18)30488-4

15   Hord, A. H., et al. (2009). "The Lost Art of the Physical Exam in Pain Medicine: A Call for Renewed Focus." *Pain Medicine,* 10(5):789–791. DOI: 10.1111/j.1526-4637.2009.00657.x.

16   Schiavenato, M., & Craig, K. D. (2010). "Pain Assessment as a Social Transaction: Beyond the 'Gold Standard'." *The Clinical Journal of Pain,* 26(8):667–676. DOI: 10.1097/AJP.0b013e3181e72507.

17   Battié, M. C., et al. (2009). "The Twin Spine Study: Contributions to a Changing View of Disc Degeneration." *The Spine Journal,* 9(1):47–59. DOI: 10.1016/j.spinee.2008.11.011.

18   Adams, M. A., & Roughley, P. J. (2006). "What Is Intervertebral Disc Degeneration, and What Causes It?" *Spine,* 31(18):2151–2161. DOI: 10.1097/01.brs.0000231761.73859.2c.

19   Urban, J. P. G., & Roberts, S. (2003). "Degeneration of the Intervertebral Disc."

Arthritis Research & Therapy, 5(3):120–130. DOI: 10.1186/ar629

20 Boos, N., et al. (2002). "Natural History of Individuals with Asymptomatic Disc Abnormalities in Magnetic Resonance Imaging: Predictors of Low Back Pain-Related Medical Consultation." *Spine*, 27(11):1143–1150. DOI: 10.1097/00007632-200205150-00006

21 Fournier DE, Kiser PK, Shoemaker JK, Battié MC, Séguin CA. Vascularization of the human intervertebral disc: A scoping review. *JOR Spine*. 2020 Sep 15;3(4):e1123. doi: 10.1002/jsp2.1123. PMID: 33392458; PMCID: PMC7770199.

22 Maciałczyk-Paprocka, K., et al. (2017). "Posture in Early Childhood: A Longitudinal Study of 3- to 6-Year-Old Children." *Journal of Physical Therapy Science*, 29(8):1395–1399. DOI: 10.1589/jpts.29.1395.

23 Gallahue, D. L., & Ozmun, J. C. (2006). "Understanding Motor Development: Infants, Children, Adolescents, Adults." *Journal of Physical Education, Recreation & Dance*

24 Payne, V. G., & Isaacs, L. D. (2017). "Human Motor Development: A Lifespan Approach." *Adapted Physical Activity Quarterly*

25 Malina, R. M., et al. (2004). "Growth, Maturation, and Physical Activity." *Human Kinetics*

26 Beunen, G., & Malina, R. M. (1988). "Growth and Physical Performance Relative to the Timing of the Adolescent Spurt." *Exercise and Sport Sciences Reviews*, 16:503-540. DOI: 10.1249/00003677-198800160-00018

27 Hirtz, P., & Starosta, W. (2002). "Sensitive and Critical Periods of Motor Coordination Development and Its Relation to Motor Learning." *Journal of Human Kinetics*, 7:19–28.

28 Massion, J. (1992). "Movement, Posture and Equilibrium: Interaction and Coordination." *Progress in Neurobiology*, 38(1):35–56. DOI: 10.1016/0301-0082(92)90034-C

Chapter 2: Revolution

1 Froud, R., et al. (2014). "A Systematic Review and Meta-Synthesis of Patients' Experiences and Perceptions of Seeking and Receiving Treatment for Chronic Low Back Pain." *Health Expectations*, 17(6):885–897.

2 Kamper, S. J., et al. (2015). "Multidisciplinary Biopsychosocial Rehabilitation for Chronic Low Back Pain: Cochrane Systematic Review and Meta-Analysis." *BMJ*, 350:h444.

3   Deyo, R. A., et al. (2009). "Overtreating Chronic Back Pain: Time to Back Off?" *Journal of the American Board of Family Medicine*, 22(1):62–68.

4   National Institutes of Health. (2023). *Back Pain Consortium (BACPAC) Research Program*. NIH HEAL Initiative

5   Froud, "Chronic Low Back Pain," 885–897.

6   Manchikanti, L., et al. (2021). "Lack of Superiority of Epidural Injections with Lidocaine with Steroids Compared to Without Steroids in Spinal Pain: A Systematic Review and Meta-Analysis." *Pain Physician*, 24(1):41–59.

7   Epidural steroid injections are not effective for patients with lumbar spinal stenosis, Steven J Atlas *BMJ* Commentary on: Friedly JL, Comstock BA, Turner JA, et al. A randomized trial of epidural glucocorticoid injections for spinal stenosis. N Engl J Med 2014;371:11–21

8   Hayden, J. A., et al. (2021). "Exercise Therapy for Chronic Low Back Pain." *Cochrane Database of Systematic Reviews*, 10(10):CD009790.

9   Cohen, S. P., et al. (2008). "Intraarticular Facet Joint Steroid Injections Are Not Effective for Chronic Low Back Pain: A Randomized Controlled Trial." *Annals of Internal Medicine*

10   Juch, J. N. S., et al. (2017). "Effect of Radiofrequency Denervation on Pain Intensity Among Patients With Chronic Low Back Pain: The Mint Randomized Clinical Trials." *JAMA*, 318(1):68–81.

11   Schwarzer, A. C., et al. (1995). "The Sacroiliac Joint in Chronic Low Back Pain." *Spine*, 20(1):31–37.

12   Moseley, G. L., & Butler, D. S. (2015). "Fifteen Years of Explaining Pain: The Past, Present, and Future." *The Journal of Pain*, 16(9):807–813.

13   Ashar, Y. K., et al. (2022). "Effect of Pain Reprocessing Therapy vs Placebo and Usual Care for Patients With Chronic Back Pain: A Randomized Clinical Trial." *JAMA Psychiatry*, 79(1):13–23.

14   Deyo RA, Dworkin SF, Amtmann D, et al. Report of the NIH Task Force on Research Standards for Chronic Low Back Pain. *Journal of Pain*. 2014;15(6):569–585.

15   Bonakdar, R., et al. (2019). "Analysis of State Insurance Coverage for Nonpharmacologic Treatment of Low Back Pain as Recommended by the American College of Physicians Guidelines." *Global Advances in Health and Medicine*, 8:1–10.

16   Freburger, J. K., et al. (2009). "The Rising Prevalence of Chronic Low Back

Pain." *Archives of Internal Medicine*, 169(3):251–258.

17 Lin, C.-W. C., et al. (2011). "Cost-effectiveness of guideline-endorsed treatments for low back pain: a systematic review." *European Spine Journal*, 20(7):1024–1038.

18 Herman, P. M., et al. (2019). "Are Nonpharmacologic Interventions for Chronic Low Back Pain More Cost Effective Than Usual Care? Proof of Concept Results from a Markov Model." *Spine*, 44(20):1456–1464.

19 Mannion, A. F., et al. (2013). "Comparison of Spinal Fusion and Nonoperative Treatment in Patients With Chronic Low Back Pain: Long-Term Follow-up of Three Randomized Controlled Trials." *Spine Journal*, 13(11):1438–1448.

20 Mirza, S. K., & Deyo, R. A. (2007). "Systematic Review of Randomized Trials Comparing Lumbar Fusion Surgery to Nonoperative Care for Chronic Back Pain." Spine, 32(7):816–823.

21 Kongsted, A., et al. (2016). "What Have We Learned From Ten Years of Trajectory Research in Low Back Pain?" *BMC Musculoskeletal Disorders*, 17:220.

22 Bonakdar, "American College of Physicians Guidelines," 1–10.

23 Manchikanti, L., et al. (2016). "Facet Joint Pain in Chronic Spinal Pain: An Evaluation of Prevalence and False-Positive Rates Using Controlled Diagnostic Blocks." *Pain Physician*, 19(2):E187–E200.

Chapter 3: Free Your Mind

1 Konstantinou, K., & Dunn, K. M. (2008). "Sciatica: Review of Epidemiological Studies and Prevalence Estimates." Spine, 33(22), 2464–2472.

2 Koes, B. W., van Tulder, M. W., & Peul, W. C. (2007). "Diagnosis and Treatment of Sciatica." *BMJ*, 334(7607), 1313–1317.

3 Cheung, K. M., Karppinen, J., Chan, D., et al. (2009). "Prevalence and Pattern of Lumbar Magnetic Resonance Imaging Changes in a Population Study of One Thousand Forty-Three Individuals." *Spine*, 34(9), 934–940.

4 Smith-Bindman, R., Kwan, M. L., Marlow, E. C., et al. (2019). "Trends in Use of Medical Imaging in US Health Care Systems and Implications for Radiology Training." *JAMA*, 322(9), 843–855.

5 Koes, van Tulder, & Peul, "Sciatica," 1313–1317.

6 Systematic Literature Review of Imaging Features of Spinal Degeneration in Asymptomatic Populations W. Brinjikji, P.H. Luetmer, B. Comstock, B.W.

Bresnahan, L.E. Chen, R.A. Deyo, S. Halabi, J.A. Turner, A.L. Avins, K. James, J.T. Wald, D.F. Kallmes and J.G. Jarvik *American Journal of Neuroradiology* April 2015, 36 (4) 811–816;

7   Masui T, Yukawa Y, Nakamura S, Kajino G, Matsubara Y, Kato F, Ishiguro N. Natural history of patients with lumbar disc herniation observed by magnetic resonance imaging for minimum 7 years. *J Spinal Disord Tech.* 2005 Apr;18(2):121-6.

8   Bogduk, N. (2005). *Clinical Anatomy of the Lumbar Spine and Sacrum.* Churchill Livingstone, 4th ed., 147–159.

9   Magnetic Resonance Imaging of the Lumbar Spine in People without Back Pain: Maureen C. Jensen, Michael N. Brant-Zawadzki, Nancy Obuchowski, Michael T. Modic, Dennis Malkasian, and Jeffrey S. Ross Published July 14, 1994 *N Engl J Med* 1994;331:69–73

10 Fullen, B. M., Doody, C., Baxter, G. D., O'Donovan, B., & O'Sullivan, K. (2019). "Examining Barriers and Facilitators to the Implementation of Best Practice Guidelines for the Management of Low Back Pain in Primary Care: A Systematic Review." *Implementation Science*, 14, 91.

11 Cohen, S. P., et al. (2020). "Pain Management Best Practices from Multispecialty Organizations During the COVID-19 Pandemic and Public Health Crises." *Pain Medicine*, 21(7), 1331–1346.

12 Citation: Maher, C., Underwood, M., & Buchbinder, R. (2017). "Non-Specific Low Back Pain." *The Lancet*, 389(10070), 736–747.

13 Dubois, M. Y., Gallagher, R. M., & Lippe, P. M. (2009). "Pain Medicine Position Paper." *Pain Medicine*, 10(6), 972–1000.

14 Moog, F. P., Karenberg, A., & Moll, F. C. (2005). "The 'Neuroanatomy' of Herophilus and Erasistratus in Context: A Historical Review." *Journal of the History of the Neurosciences*, 14(3), 223–234.

15 Pearce, J. M. S. (2012). "Galen and His Contributions to Neurology." *Journal of Neurological Sciences*, 317(1-2), 1-3.

16 Perl, E. R. (2007). "Ideas About Pain, a Historical View." *Nature Reviews Neuroscience*, 8(1), 71–79.

17 Melzack, R., & Wall, P. D. (1965). "Pain Mechanisms: A New Theory." *Science*, 150(3699), 971–979.

18 Tauben, D. J., & Loeser, J. D. (2013). "Pain Education at the University of Washington School of Medicine." *The Journal of Pain*, 14(5), 431–437.

19 Steinberg, E. P., & Martin, B. I. (1986). "The Diffusion of Magnetic Resonance Imaging Scanners in the United States." *Journal of the American Medical Association*, 255(11), 1466–1470.

20 Overington, J. P., Al-Lazikani, B., & Hopkins, A. L. (2006). "How Many Drug Targets Are There?" *Nature Reviews Drug Discovery*, 5(12), 993–996.

21 Chou, R., & Huffman, L. H. (2007). "Nonpharmacologic Therapies for Acute and Chronic Low Back Pain: A Review of the Evidence for an American Pain Society/American College of Physicians Clinical Practice Guideline." *Annals of Internal Medicine*, 147(7), 492–504.

22 Deer, T. R., Mekhail, N., Provenzano, D., et al. (2014). "The Appropriate Use of Neurostimulation of the Spinal Cord and Peripheral Nervous System for the Treatment of Chronic Pain and Ischemic Diseases: The Neuromodulation Appropriateness Consensus Committee." *Neuromodulation*, 17(6), 515–550.

23 Bushnell, M. C., Čeko, M., & Low, L. A. (2013). "Cognitive and Emotional Control of Pain and Its Disruption in Chronic Pain." *Nature Reviews Neuroscience*, 14(7), 502–511.

24 Meldrum, M. L. (2003). "A Capsule History of Pain Management." *JAMA*, 290(18), 2470–2475.

25 Bogduk, N. (2009). "On the Definitions and Physiology of Back Pain, Referred Pain, and Radicular Pain." *Pain*, 147(1-3), 17–19.

26 Bonica, J. J. (1953). *The Management of Pain*. Lea & Febiger, 532–560.

27 Kapural, L., Deer, T. R., & Amirdelfan, K. (2022). "Advances in Pain Medicine: A Review of New Technologies." *Current Pain and Headache Reports*, 26(8), 605–615.

28 Meldrum, M. L. (2003). "A Capsule History of Pain Management." *JAMA*, 290(18), 2470–2475.

29 Fishman, S. M., Young, H. M., Lucas Arwood, E., et al. (2013). "Core Competencies for Pain Management: Results of an Interprofessional Consensus Summit." *Pain Medicine*, 14(7), 971–981.

30 DePalma, M. J., Ketchum, J. M., & Saullo, T. (2011). "What Is the Source of Chronic Low Back Pain and Does Age Play a Role?" *Pain Medicine*, 12(2), 224–233.

31 Deer, Mekhail, Provenzano, et al, "Neuromodulation Appropriateness," 515–550.

32 Manchikanti, L., Kaye, A. D., Soin, A., et al. (2021). "Lack of Superiority of Epi-

dural Injections with Lidocaine with Steroids Compared to Without Steroids in Spinal Pain: A Systematic Review and Meta-Analysis." *Pain Physician*, 24(1), 41–59.

33 Chou, R., Atlas, S. J., Stanos, S. P., & Rosenquist, R. W. (2009). "Nonsurgical Interventional Therapies for Low Back Pain: A Review of the Evidence for an American Pain Society Clinical Practice Guideline." *Spine*, 34(10), 1078–1093.

34 Bogduk, N. (2005). "Diagnostic Blocks: A Truth Serum for Pain." *Clinical Journal of Pain*, 21(5), 409–414.

35 Martin, H. D., Kelly, B. T., Leunig, M., et al. (2006). "The Pattern and Technique in the Clinical Evaluation of the Adult Hip: The Common Physical Examination Tests of Hip Specialists." *Journal of Arthroscopy and Related Surgery*, 22(10),

36 Hegedus, E. J., Goode, A. P., Cook, C. E., et al. (2012). "Which Physical Examination Tests Provide Clinicians with the Most Value When Examining the Shoulder? Update of a Systematic Review With Meta-Analysis of Individual Tests." *British Journal of Sports Medicine*, 46(14), 964–978

37 Jackson, J. L., O'Malley, P. G., & Kroenke, K. (2003). "Evaluation of Acute Knee Pain in Primary Care." *Annals of Internal Medicine*, 139(7), 575–588.

38 Cohen SP, Bhaskar A, Bhatia A, et al. Consensus practice guidelines on interventions for lumbar facet joint pain from a Multispecialty, International Working group. Regional Anesthesia *Pain Medicine*. 2020;45(6):424–467.

39 Manchikanti L, Kaye A, Soin A, et al. Comprehensive Evidence-Based Guidelines for Facet Joint Interventions in the Management of Chronic Spinal Pain: American Society of Interventional Pain Physicians (ASIPP) Guidelines Facet Joint Interventions 2020 Guidelines. *J Pain Physician*. 2020;23(3S):S1–S127.

40 Boswell MV, Manchikanti L, Kaye AD, et al. A Best-Evidence Systematic Appraisal of the Diagnostic Accuracy and Utility of Facet (Zygapophysial) Joint Injections in Chronic Spinal Pain. *Pain Physician*. 2015;18(4):E497533.

41 Sacroiliac joint pain after multiple-segment lumbar fusion: a long-term observational study-Non-fused sacrum vs. fused sacrum, Eiki Unoki et al Spine surgery relay. *Res*. 2017 Dec 20

42 Sacroiliac joint pain after lumbar fusion. A study with anesthetic blocks J. Y. Maigne et al *Europ. Sine J* Sept 2005

43 Petroianu, A. (2012). "Diagnosis of Acute Appendicitis." *International Journal of Surgery*, 10(3), 115–119.

44 Hooton, T. M. (2012). "Uncomplicated Urinary Tract Infection." *New England Journal of Medicine*, 366(11), 1028–1037.

45 Centers for Medicare & Medicaid Services (CMS). (2021). "Local Coverage Determination (LCD): Facet Joint Interventions for Pain Management (L38841)." Medicare Coverage Database.

46 Bogduk, "Truth Serum," 409–414.

47 McCormick, Z. L., Marshall, B., Walker, J., McCarthy, R., & Walega, D. R. (2015). "Long-Term Function, Pain and Medication Use Outcomes of Radiofrequency Ablation for Lumbar Facet Syndrome." *International Journal of Anesthesia and Anesthesiology*

48 Dreyfuss P, Stout A, Aprill C, Pollei S, Johnson B, Bogduk N. The significance of multifidus atrophy after successful radiofrequency neurotomy for low back pain. *PM R*. 2009 Aug;1(8):719–22

49 Wilson, J. C., McEvoy, L. K., & Jain, S. (2008). "Systemic Effects of Local Corticosteroid Injections: A Review." *Journal of Clinical Rheumatology*, 14(5), 287–292.

50 Manchikanti, L., Cash, K. A., McManus, C. D., et al. (2015). "Do Epidural Injections Provide Short- and Long-Term Relief for Lumbar Disc Herniation? A Systematic Review." *Pain Physician*, 18(1), 1–23.

51 AlAli, K. F. (2023). "Unnecessary Spine Surgery: Can We Solve This Ongoing Conundrum?" *Frontiers in Surgery*, 10, 1270975.

52 Cohen, S. P. (2005). "Sacroiliac Joint Pain: A Comprehensive Review of Anatomy, Diagnosis, and Treatment." *Anesthesia & Analgesia*, 101(5), 1440–1453.

53 Kamali, F., & Shokri, E. (2012). "The Effect of Two Manipulative Therapy Techniques and Their Outcome in Patients With Sacroiliac Joint Syndrome." *Journal of Bodywork and Movement Therapies*, 16(1), 29–35.

54 Polly, D. W., & Cher, D. J. (2017). "Sacroiliac Fusion: Another 'Magic Bullet' Destined for Disrepute." *Neurosurgery Clinics of North America*, 28(3), 313–317.

55 Hayden, J. A., Ellis, J., Ogilvie, R., et al. (2021). "Exercise Therapy for Chronic Low Back Pain." *Cochrane Database of Systematic Reviews*, 10(10), CD009790

56 Kamper, S. J., Apeldoorn, A. T., Chiarotto, A., et al. (2015). "Multidisciplinary Biopsychosocial Rehabilitation for Chronic Low Back Pain: Cochrane Systematic Review and Meta-Analysis." *BMJ*, 350, h444.

57 Machado, L. A. C., Kamper, S. J., Herbert, R. D., Maher, C. G., & McAuley, J. H. (2009). "Analgesic Effects of Treatments for Non-Specific Low Back Pain:

A Meta-Analysis of Placebo-Controlled Randomized Trials." *Rheumatology*, 48(5), 520–527.

58 Wand, B. M., Bird, C., McAuley, J. H., et al. (2004). "Early Intervention for Acute Low Back Pain Patients: Does It Matter? Randomized Controlled Trial of General Exercise vs. Motor Control Exercise." *Spine*, 29(19), 2090–2100.

59 Hayden, J. A., Ellis, J., Ogilvie, R., et al. (2021). "Exercise Therapy for Chronic Low Back Pain." *Cochrane Database of Systematic Reviews*, 10(10), CD009790.

60 Smith, B. E., Littlewood, C., & May, S. (2014). "An Update of Stabilisation Exercises for Low Back Pain: A Systematic Review With Meta-Analysis." *BMC Musculoskeletal Disorders*, 15, 416.

61 McGill, S. M. (2001). "Low Back Stability: From Formal Description to Issues for Performance and Rehabilitation." *Exercise and Sport Sciences Reviews*, 29(1), 26–31.

62 Hodges, P. W., & Richardson, C. A. (1997). "Contraction of the Abdominal Muscles Associated With Movement of the Lower Limb." *Physical Therapy*, 77(2), 132–142.

63 Manchikanti, Cash, McManus, et al, "Lumbar Disc Herniation," 1–23.

64 Baber, Z., & Erdek, M. A. (2016). "Failed Back Surgery Syndrome: Current Perspectives." *Journal of Pain Research*, 9, 979–987.

65 Miekisiak, G. (2023). "Failed Back Surgery Syndrome: No Longer a Surgeon's Defeat—A Narrative Review." *Journal of Clinical Medicine*, 12(13), 4476.

66 Kongsted, A., Kent, P., Hestbaek, L., & Vach, W. (2016). "What Have We Learned From Ten Years of Trajectory Research in Low Back Pain?" *BMC Musculoskeletal Disorders*, 17, 220.

67 Hashmi, J. A., Baliki, M. N., Huang, L., et al. (2013). "Shape Shifting Pain: Chronification of Back Pain Shifts Brain Representation From Nociceptive to Emotional Circuits." *Brain*, 136(9), 2751–2768.

Chapter 4: Your Body Guitar

1 Casazza BA, Young JL. Back pain. In: *StatPearls*. StatPearls Publishing; 2023. PMID: 29262063.

2 DePalma MJ, Ketchum JM, Saullo T. What is the source of chronic low back pain and does age play a role? *Pain Med*. 2011;12(2):224–233. doi:10.1111/j.1526-4637.2010.01045.x

3   Cheung KMC, Karppinen J, Chan D, et al. Prevalence and pattern of lumbar magnetic resonance imaging changes in a population study of one thousand forty-three individuals. *Spine* (Phila Pa 1976). 2009;34(9):934–940. doi:10.1097/BRS.0b013e3181a01b3f

4   Qaseem A, Wilt TJ, McLean RM, et al. Noninvasive treatments for acute, subacute, and chronic low back pain: a clinical practice guideline from the American College of Physicians. *Ann Intern Med.* 2017;166(7):514–530. doi:10.7326/M16-2367

5   Lund JP, Donga R, Widmer CG, Stohler CS. The pain-adaptation model: a discussion of the relationship between chronic musculoskeletal pain and motor activity. Scand J *Work Environ Health.* 1991;17(1):13–20. doi:10.5271/sjweh.1740

6   Solomonow M. Time dependent spine stability: the wise old man and the six blind elephants. *Clin Biomech* (Bristol, Avon). 2011;26(3):219–222. doi:10.1016/j.clinbiomech.2010.10.005

7   Jaumard NV, Welch WC, Winkelstein BA. Spinal facet joint biomechanics and mechanotransduction in normal, injury and degenerative conditions. *Annu Rev Biomed Eng.* 2011;13:325–353. doi:10.1146/annurev-bioeng-071910-124658

8   Bogduk N. *Clinical Anatomy of the Lumbar Spine and Sacrum.* 4th ed. Churchill Livingstone; 2005.

9   White AA, Panjabi MM. *Clinical Biomechanics of the Spine.* 2nd ed. Lippincott Williams & Wilkins; 1990.

10 Punchard NA, Whelan CJ, Adcock I. *The Journal of Inflammation: a new journal for a new era.* J Inflamm (Lond). 2004;1:1. doi:10.1186/1476-9255-1-1

11 Medzhitov R. Origin and physiological roles of inflammation. *Nature.* 2008;454(7203):428–435. doi:10.1038/nature07201

12 Hodges PW, Tucker K. Moving differently in pain: a new theory to explain the adaptation to pain. *Pain.* 2011;152(3 Suppl):S90–S98. doi:10.1016/j.pain.2010.10.027

13 Hopkins JT, Ingersoll CD. Arthrogenic muscle inhibition: a limiting factor in joint rehabilitation. *J Sport Rehabil.* 2000;9(2):135–159. doi:10.1123/jsr.9.2.135

14 McGill SM. Low back stability: from formal description to issues for performance and rehabilitation. *Exerc Sport Sci Rev.* 2001;29(1):26–31. doi:10.1097/00003677-200101000-00006

15 MacDonald DA, Moseley GL, Hodges PW. The lumbar multifidus: does the evidence support clinical beliefs? *Man Ther.* 2006;11(4):254–263. doi:10.1016/j.

math.2006.02.004

16 Kim CW, Gottschalk LJ, Eng C, et al. The multifidus muscle is the strongest stabilizer of the lumbar spine. *Spine J.* 2007;7(5):76S. doi:10.1016/j.spinee.2007.07.187

17 Hodges PW, Gandevia SC. Changes in intra-abdominal pressure during postural and respiratory activation of the human diaphragm. *J Appl Physiol* (1985). 2000;89(3):967–976. doi:10.1152/jappl.2000.89.3.967

18 Kolar P, Sulc J, Kyncl M, et al. Postural function of the diaphragm in persons with and without chronic low back pain. *J Orthop Sports Phys Ther.* 2012;42(4):352–362. doi:10.2519/jospt.2012.3830

19 McGill SM, Hughson RL, Parks K. The psoas major and lumbar spine stability: a biomechanical analysis. *Clin Biomech* (Bristol, Avon). 1996;11(5):257–263. doi:10.1016/0268-0033(96)00003-3

20 Neumann DA. Kinesiology of the hip: a focus on muscular actions. *J Orthop Sports Phys Ther.* 2010;40(2):82–94. doi:10.2519/jospt.2010.3025

21 Ingber RS. Iliopsoas myofascial dysfunction: a treatable cause of "failed" low back syndrome. *Arch Phys Med Rehabil.* 1989;70(5):382–386. PMID: 2524206

22 Vernon H, Meschino J, Naiman J. Inversion therapy: a study of physiological effects. *J Can Chiropr Assoc.* 1985;29(3):135-140. PMID: 2933387

23 Lam OT, Strenger DM, Chan-Fee M, et al. Effectiveness of the McKenzie Method of Mechanical Diagnosis and Therapy for treating low back pain: literature review with meta-analysis. *J Orthop Sports Phys Ther.* 2018;48(6):476–490. doi:10.2519/jospt.2018.7562

24 Pickar JG, Bolton PS. Spinal manipulative therapy and somatosensory activation. *J Electromyogr Kinesiol.* 2012;22(5):785–794. doi:10.1016/j.jelekin.2012.01.015

25 Kisiel J. Tame Your Hip Flexors With the Egoscue Tower. *The Pain Free Athlete*; 2014.

26 Sarno JE. *Healing Back Pain: The Mind-Body Connection.* Warner Books; 1991.

27 Ingber RS. Iliopsoas myofascial dysfunction: a treatable cause of "failed" low back syndrome. *Arch Phys Med Rehabil.* 1989;70(5):382–386. PMID: 2524206

28 Whiler L, Fong M, Kim S, et al. Gluteus medius and minimus muscle structure, strength, and function in healthy adults: brief report. *Physiother Can.* 2017;69(3):212–216. doi:10.3138/ptc.2016-16

29 Nakamura J, Kariyama Y, Nakayama S, et al. Impacts of external rotators and the ischiofemoral ligament on preventing excessive internal hip rotation: a cadaveric study. *J Orthop Surg Res.* 2022;17(1):4. doi:10.1186/s13018-021-02895-7

30 Gottschalk F, Kourosh S, Leveau B. The functional anatomy of the gluteus medius and minimus muscles and their relationship to hip joint stability. *J Anat.* 1989;164:163–174. PMID: 2606798

31 Boonstra TW, Daffertshofer A, Beek PJ. Revisiting Leonardo on muscles: intimations of mathematical biology and biomechanics. *Biol Theory.* 2023;18:156–169. doi:10.1007/s13752-023-00436-8

32 Cresswell AG, Oddsson L, Thorstensson A. The influence of sudden perturbations on trunk muscle activity and intra-abdominal pressure while standing. *Exp Brain Res.* 1994;98(2):336–341. doi:10.1007/BF00228421

33 Freeman MD, Woodham MA, Woodham AW. The role of the lumbar multifidus in chronic low back pain: a review. *PM R.* 2010;2(2):142–146. doi:10.1016/j.pmrj.2009.11.006

34 Hides J, Gilmore C, Stanton W, Bohlscheid E. Multifidus size and symmetry among chronic LBP and healthy asymptomatic subjects. *Man Ther.* 2008;13(1):43–49. doi:10.1016/j.math.2006.07.017

35 Kiapour A, Joukar A, Elgafy H, Erbulut DU, Agarwal AK, Goel VK. Biomechanics of the sacroiliac joint: anatomy, function, biomechanics, sexual dimorphism, and causes of pain. *Int J Spine Surg.* 2020;14(Suppl 1):S3–S13. doi:10.14444/6077

36 Vleeming A, Schuenke MD, Masi AT, Carreiro JE, Danneels L, Willard FH. The sacroiliac joint: an overview of its anatomy, function and potential clinical implications. *J Anat.* 2012;221(6):537–567. doi:10.1111/j.1469-7580.2012.01519.x

37 Falowski S, Sayed D. Sacroiliac joint dysfunction: diagnosis and treatment. *Am Fam Physician.* 2022;105(3):251–258. PMID: 35289566

38 Wong M, Sinkler MA, Kiel J. Sacroiliac joint injury. In: *StatPearls.* StatPearls Publishing; 2023. PMID: 33085281

39 Verywell Health. Facet joint disorders and pain: symptoms, treatment, and more. October 13, 2023. Accessed February 28, 2025. https://www.verywellhealth.com/facet-joint-pain-7560142

40 Spine-health. Symptoms and diagnosis of facet joint disorders. June 23, 2020. Accessed February 28, 2025. https://www.spine-health.com/conditions/spine-anatomy/symptoms-and-diagnosis-facet-joint-disorders

41 Hauser RA, Steilen-Matias D. Sacroiliac joint dysfunction symptoms and treatment options. *Caring Medical.* 2024. Accessed February 28, 2025. https://www.caringmedical.com/prolotherapy-news/sacroiliac-joint-dysfunction-treatment/

42 SpineUniverse. Lower back pain symptoms, diagnosis, and treatment. March 10, 2021. Accessed February 28, 2025. https://www.spineuniverse.com/conditions/back-pain/low-back-pain/low-back-pain-symptoms-diagnosis-treatment

43 SpineUniverse. Herniated discs: definition, progression, and diagnosis. March 10, 2021. Accessed February 28, 2025. https://www.spineuniverse.com/conditions/herniated-disc/herniated-discs-definition-progression-diagnosis

44 Newcastle Sports Medicine. Trochanteric bursitis and gluteal tendinopathy–assessment and treatment options. October 29, 2018. Accessed February 28, 2025. https://newcastlesportsmedicine.com.au/trochanteric-bursitis-gluteal-tendinopathy-assessment-treatment-options/

45 Johns Hopkins Medicine. Iliotibial band syndrome. April 30, 2024. Accessed February 28, 2025. https://www.hopkinsmedicine.org/health/conditions-and-diseases/iliotibial-band-syndrome

46 Bayram S, Barman H. Piriformis syndrome as an overlooked cause of pain in a patient with axial spondyloarthritis: a case report. *Clin Med* (Lond). 2020;20(3):e18–e19. doi:10.7861/clinmed.2020-0065

47 Mya Care. Piriformis syndrome & herniated disc: similarities and differences. July 25, 2024. Accessed February 28, 2025. https://myacare.com/blog/piriformis-syndrome-herniated-disc-similarities-and-differences

48 Hauser RA, Steilen-Matias D. Piriformis syndrome and sciatica pain. Caring Medical. 2024. Accessed February 28, 2025. https://www.caringmedical.com/prolotherapy-news/piriformis-syndrome-sciatica-pain/

49 Wong M, Sinkler MA, Kiel J. Piriformis syndrome. In: *StatPearls.* StatPearls Publishing; 2023. PMID: 29493940

50 Callister WD, Rethwisch DG. *Materials Science and Engineering: An Introduction.* 10th ed. Wiley; 2018.

51 González-Alonso J, Crandall CG, Johnson JM. Heat production in human skeletal muscle at the onset of intense dynamic exercise. *J Physiol.* 2000;524(Pt 2):603–615. doi:10.1111/j.1469-7793.2000.t01-1-00603.x

52 Jay GD, Waller KA. The biology of lubricin: near frictionless joint motion. *Matrix Biol.* 2014;39:17–24. doi:10.1016/j.matbio.2014.08.008

53 Knight MM, Levick JR. The effect of joint movement on the temperature of synovial fluid in the rabbit knee. *J Physiol.* 1983;343:335–345. doi:10.1113/jphysiol.1983.sp014895

54 Urban, J. P. G., & Roberts, S. (2003). "Degeneration of the Intervertebral Disc." *Arthritis Research & Therapy*, 5(3):120–130. DOI: 10.1186/ar629

55 Boos, N., et al. (2002). "Natural History of Individuals with Asymptomatic Disc Abnormalities in Magnetic Resonance Imaging: Predictors of Low Back Pain-Related Medical Consultation." *Spine*, 27(11):1143–1150. DOI: 10.1097/00007632-200205150-00006

56 Fournier DE, Kiser PK, Shoemaker JK, Battié MC, Séguin CA. Vascularization of the human intervertebral disc: A scoping review. *JOR Spine.* 2020 Sep 15;3(4):e1123. doi: 10.1002/jsp2.1123. PMID: 33392458; PMCID: PMC7770199.

57 Raj PP. Intervertebral disc: anatomy-physiology-pathophysiology-treatment. *Pain Pract.* 2008;8(1):18–44. doi:10.1111/j.1533-2500.2007.00159.x

58 Fardon DF, Milette PC. Nomenclature and classification of lumbar disc pathology: recommendations of the Combined Task Forces of the North American Spine Society, American Society of Spine Radiology, and American Society of Neuroradiology. *Spine* (Phila Pa 1976). 2001;26(5):E93–E113. doi:10.1097/00007632-200103010-00006

59 Casey E. Natural history of radiculopathy. *Phys Med Rehabil Clin N Am.* 2012;23(1):1–12. doi:10.1016/j.pmr.2011.11.001

60 Ropper AH, Zafonte RD. Sciatica. *N Engl J Med.* 2015;372(13):1240–1248. doi:10.1056/NEJMra1410151

61 Amin RM, Andrade NS, Neuman BJ. Lumbar disc herniation. *Curr Rev Musculoskelet Med.* 2017;10(4):507–516. doi:10.1007/s12178-017-9441-4

62 Brinjikji W, Luetmer PH, Comstock B, et al. Systematic literature review of imaging features of spinal degeneration in asymptomatic populations. *AJNR Am J Neuroradiol.* 2015;36(4):811–816. doi:10.3174/ajnr.A4173

63 Peng BG. Pathophysiology, diagnosis, and treatment of discogenic low back pain. *World J Orthop.* 2013;4(2):42–52. doi:10.5312/wjo.v4.i2.42

64 Falco FJE, Manchikanti L, Datta S, et al. An updated review of diagnostic and therapeutic spinal interventions for chronic low back pain. *Pain Physician.* 2021;24:S1–S53. PMID: 34704706

65 Manchikanti L, Sanapati MR, Pampati V, et al. Lumbar epidural injections in the treatment of chronic low back pain: a systematic review and update. *Pain*

Physician. 2021;24:E645–E689. PMID: 34704708

Chapter 5: Change Your Constitution

1   Schiaffino, S., & Reggiani, C. (2011). "Fiber types in mammalian skeletal muscles." *Physiological Reviews,* 91(4), 1447–1531. doi:10.1152/physrev.00031.2010

2   Seynnes, O. R., de Boer, M., & Narici, M. V. (2007). "Early skeletal muscle hypertrophy and architectural changes in response to high-intensity resistance training." *Journal of Applied Physiology,* 102(1), 368–373. doi:10.1152/japplphysiol.00789.2006

3   Mujika, I., & Padilla, S. (2000). "Detraining: Loss of training-induced physiological and performance adaptations. Part I: Short term insufficient training stimulus." *Sports Medicine,* 30(2), 79–87. doi:10.2165/00007256-200030020-00002

4   Staron, R. S., et al. (1991). "Skeletal muscle adaptations during early phase of heavy-resistance training in men and women." *Journal of Applied Physiology,* 70(3), 1246–1254. doi:10.1152/jappl.1991.70.3.1246

5   Holloszy, J. O., & Coyle, E. F. (1984). "Adaptations of skeletal muscle to endurance exercise and their metabolic consequences." *Journal of Applied Physiology,* 56(4), 831–838. doi:10.1152/jappl.1984.56.4.831

6   Romanul, F. C. A. (1965). "Capillary supply and metabolism of muscle fibers." *Archives of Neurology,* 12(5), 497–509. doi:10.1001/archneur.1965.00460290013003

7   Saltin, B., & Gollnick, P. D. (1983). "Skeletal muscle adaptability: Significance for metabolism and performance." *Handbook of Physiology: Skeletal Muscle,* 555–631.

8   Hawley, J. A., et al. (2014). "Integrative biology of exercise." *Cell,* 159(4), 738–749. doi:10.1016/j.cell.2014.10.029

9   Laughlin, M. H., & Roseguini, B. (2008). "Mechanisms for exercise training-induced increases in skeletal muscle blood flow capacity: Differences with interval sprint training versus aerobic endurance training." *Journal of Physiology and Pharmacology,* 59(Suppl 7), 71–88. PMID: 19258658

10 Olfert, I. M., & Birot, O. (2011). "Molecular and cellular mechanisms of skeletal muscle angiogenesis." *Microcirculation,* 18(6), 452–462. doi:10.1111/j.1549-8719.2011.00107.x

11 Prior, B. M., et al. (2004). "What makes vessels grow with exercise training?" *Journal of Applied Physiology,* 97(3), 1119–1128. doi:10.1152/jap-

plphysiol.00035.2004

12 Roudier, E., et al. (2012). "Endurance training in a rat model of metabolic syndrome enhances muscle angiogenesis through a VEGF-independent pathway." *Microcirculation*, 19(4), 336–346. doi:10.1111/j.1549-8719.2012.00168.x

13 Houston, M. E., et al. (1979). "Muscle performance, morphology and metabolic capacity during strength training and detraining: A one leg model." *European Journal of Applied Physiology and Occupational Physiology*, 41(4), 261–271. doi:10.1007/BF00429743

14 Ohira M, Hanada H, Kawano F, Ishihara A, Nonaka I, Ohira Y. Regulation of the properties of rat hind limb muscles following gravitational unloading. *Jpn J Physiol*. 2002 Jun;52(3):235–45. doi: 10.2170/jjphysiol.52.235. PMID: 12230800.

15 Fitts, R. H., et al. (2000). "The deleterious effects of bed rest on human skeletal muscle fibers are exacerbated by aging." *Journal of Applied Physiology*, 89(5), 1715–1725. doi:10.1152/jappl.2000.89.5.1715

16 Wilson, J. M., et al. (2012). "The effects of endurance, strength, and power training on muscle fiber type shifting." *Journal of Strength and Conditioning Research*, 26(6), 1724–1729. doi:10.1519/JSC.0b013e318234eb6f

17 Ahmetov, I. I., & Fedotovskaya, O. N. (2015). "Current progress in sports genomics." *Advances in Clinical Chemistry*, 70, 247–314. doi:10.1016/bs.acc.2015.03.003

18 Campos, G. E. R., et al. (2002). "Muscular adaptations in response to three different resistance-training regimens: Specificity of repetition maximum training zones." *European Journal of Applied Physiology*, 88(1–2), 50–60. doi:10.1007/s00421-002-0681-6

19 Proske, U., & Gandevia, S. C. (2012). "The proprioceptive senses: Their roles in signaling body shape, body position and movement, and muscle force." *Physiological Reviews*, 92(4), 1651–1697. doi:10.1152/physrev.00048.2011

20 Kröger, S., & Watkins, B. (2021). "Muscle spindle function in healthy and diseased muscle." *Skeletal Muscle*, 11(1), 3. doi:10.1186/s13395-020-00258-x

21 Hodges, P. W., & Richardson, C. A. (1997). "Contraction of the abdominal muscles associated with movement of the lower limb." *Physical Therapy*, 77(2), 132–142. doi:10.1093/ptj/77.2.132

22 McGill, S. M., et al. (2003). "Coordination of muscle activity and intra-abdominal pressure during lifting and stabilizing challenges." *Journal of Electromyography and Kinesiology*, 13(5), 463–475. doi:10.1016/S1050-6411(03)00061-0

23 Cholewicki, J., & McGill, S. M. (1996). "Mechanical stability of the in vivo lumbar spine: Implications for injury and chronic low back pain." *Clinical Bio-mechanics,* 11(1), 1–15. doi:10.1016/0268-0033(95)00035-6

24 Schiaffino & Reggiani, "Skeletal muscles," 1447–1531. doi:10.1152/physrev.00031.2010

25 LeBlanc, A., et al. (2000). "Muscle volume, strength, endurance, and exercise loads during 6-month missions in space." *Aviation, Space, and Environmental Medicine,* 71(9 Suppl), A91–A104. PMID: 10993313

26 G Antonutto, C Capelli, M Girardis, P Zamparo, P E di Prampero Effects of microgravity on maximal power of lower limbs during very short efforts in humans PMID: 9887117 DOI: 10.1152/jappl.1999.86.1.85 *J Appl Physiol* (1985) 1999 Jan;86(1):85–92. doi: 10.1152/jappl.1999.86.1.85

27 Kandel, E. R., et al. (Eds.). (2013). *Principles of Neural Science* (5th ed.), Chapter 49: "The Autonomic Nervous System and the Hypothalamus." McGraw-Hill.

28 Panjabi, M. M. (1992). "The stabilizing system of the spine. Part I. Function, dysfunction, adaptation, and enhancement." *Journal of Spinal Disorders,* 5(4), 383–389. doi:10.1097/00002517-199212000-00001

29 Tsao, H., & Hodges, P. W. (2008). "Persistence of improvements in postural strategies following motor control training in people with recurrent low back pain." *Journal of Electromyography and Kinesiology,* 18(4), 559–567. doi:10.1016/j.jelekin.2006.10.012

30 Jänig, W. (2006). "The integrative action of the autonomic nervous system: Neurobiology of homeostasis." Cambridge University Press. doi:10.1017/CBO9780511541667

31 Juker, D., et al. (1998). "Quantitative intramuscular myoelectric activity of lumbar portions of psoas and the abdominal wall during a wide variety of tasks." *Medicine & Science in Sports & Exercise,* 30(2), 301–310. doi:10.1097/00005768-199802000-00019

32 Cholewicki, J., et al. (2002). "Delayed trunk muscle reflex responses increase the risk of low back injuries." *Spine,* 27(24), 2765–2770. doi:10.1097/00007632-200212150-00006

33 Panjabi, "Function, dysfunction, adaptation, and enhancement," 383–389. doi:10.1097/00002517-199212000-00001

34 McGill, S. M. (2001). "Low back stability: From formal description to issues for performance and rehabilitation." *Exercise and Sport Sciences Reviews,* 29(1), 26–31. doi:10.1097/00003677-200101000-00006

35 Cresswell, A. G., & Thorstensson, A. (1994). "Changes in intra-abdominal pressure, trunk muscle activation and force during isokinetic lifting and lowering." *European Journal of Applied Physiology and Occupational Biomechanics, 68*(4), 315–321. doi:10.1007/BF00843736

36 Kolar, P., et al. (2012). "Postural function of the diaphragm in persons with and without chronic low back pain." *Journal of Orthopaedic & Sports Physical Therapy, 42*(4), 352–362. doi:10.2519/jospt.2012.3830

37 Hodges, P. W., & Moseley, G. L. (2003). "Pain and motor control of the lumbo-pelvic region: Effect and possible mechanisms." *Journal of Electromyography and Kinesiology, 13*(4), 361–370. doi:10.1016/S1050-6411(03)00042-7

38 Panjabi, M. M. (1992). "The stabilizing system of the spine. Part II. Neutral zone and instability hypothesis." *Journal of Spinal Disorders, 5*(4), 390–397. doi:10.1097/00002517-199212000-00002

39 Sapolsky, R. M. (2004). "Organismal stress and the hypothalamic-pituitary-adrenal axis." *Annals of the New York Academy of Sciences, 1018*(1), 192–198. doi:10.1196/annals.1296.022

40 Kapreli, E., et al. (2009). "Respiratory dysfunction in chronic neck and back pain patients: A pilot study." *Manual Therapy, 14*(5), 528–533. doi:10.1016/j.math.2008.09.002

41 Kibler, W. B., et al. (2006). "The role of core stability in athletic function." *Sports Medicine, 36*(3), 189–198. doi:10.2165/00007256-200636030-00001

42 Piek, J. P., et al. (2008). "The relationship between motor coordination and physical fitness in children." *Developmental Medicine & Child Neurology, 50*(6), 412–417. doi:10.1111/j.1469-8749.2008.03014.x

43 Malina, R. M., et al. (2004). "Growth, maturation, and physical activity." *Human Kinetics*, Chapter 11: "Motor Development and Performance." doi:10.5040/9781492596820

44 Horak, F. B. (2006). "Postural orientation and equilibrium: What do we need to know about neural control of balance to prevent falls?" *Age and Ageing, 35*(Suppl 2), ii7–ii11. doi:10.1093/ageing/afl077

45 Seidler, R. D., et al. (2010). "Motor control and aging: Links to age-related brain structural, functional, and biochemical effects." *Neuroscience & Biobehavioral Reviews, 34*(5), 721–733. doi:10.1016/j.neubiorev.2009.10.005

46 Spirduso, W. W., et al. (2005). "Physical activity, aging, and motor skill performance." *Exercise and Sport Sciences Reviews, 33*(1), 19–24. doi:10.1097/00003677-200501000-00005

47 Lieber, R. L. (2002). *Skeletal Muscle Structure, Function, and Plasticity* (2nd ed.), Chapter 3: "Muscle Mechanics." Lippincott Williams & Wilkins.

48 Stecco, C., et al. (2008). "The role of fascia in muscle coordination and joint stability." *Journal of Bodywork and Movement Therapies*, 12(3), 225–233. doi:10.1016/j.jbmt.2008.04.035

49 Willard, F. H., et al. (2012). "The thoracolumbar fascia: Anatomy, function and clinical considerations." *Journal of Anatomy*, 221(6), 507–536. doi:10.1111/j.1469-7580.2012.01511.x

50 Schleip, R., et al. (2005). "Active fascial contractility: Fascia may be able to contract in a smooth muscle-like manner and thereby influence musculoskeletal dynamics." *Medical Hypotheses*, 65(2), 273–277. doi:10.1016/j.mehy.2005.03.005

51 Gribble, P. A., & Hertel, J. (2004). "Effect of lower-extremity muscle fatigue on postural control." *Archives of Physical Medicine and Rehabilitation*, 85(4), 589–592. doi:10.1016/j.apmr.2003.06.031

52 Sah, N., et al. (2004). "Effect of anesthesia on muscle tone and movement." *Anesthesia & Analgesia*, 98(4), 1042–1047. doi:10.1213/01.ANE.0000105876.59219. FC

53 van Dieën, J. H., et al. (2003). "Trunk muscle recruitment patterns in patients with low back pain enhance the stability of the lumbar spine." *Spine*, 28(8), 834–841. doi:10.1097/01.BRS.0000058932.15331.3A

54 Schleip, "Musculoskeletal dynamics," 273–277. doi:10.1016/j.mehy.2005.03.005

55 Butler, D. S., & Moseley, G. L. (2003). *Explain Pain.* Noigroup Publications.

56 Baliki, M. N., et al. (2008). "Chronic pain and the emotional brain: Specific brain activity associated with spontaneous fluctuations of intensity of chronic back pain." *Journal of Neuroscience*, 26(47), 12165–12173. doi:10.1523/JNEUROSCI.3576-06.2008

57 Melzack R, Wall PD. Pain Mechanisms: A New Theory. *Science* 150(3699) 971-9 Nov 1965

58 Apkarian, A. V., et al. (2011). "Pain and the brain: Specificity and plasticity of the brain in clinical chronic pain." *Pain*, 152(3 Suppl), S49–S64. doi:10.1016/j.pain.2010.11.010

59 Solomonow, M., et al. (1998). "The ligamento-muscular stabilizing system of the spine." *Spine*, 23(23), 2552–2562. doi:10.1097/00007632-199812010-00014

60 Ralphs, J. R., & Benjamin, M. (1994). "The joint capsule: Structure, composition, ageing and disease." *Journal of Anatomy*, 184(Pt 3), 503–509. PMCID:

PMC1259986

61 Hill, C. L., et al. (2001). "The role of the joint capsule in the stability of the elbow joint." *Journal of Bone and Joint Surgery*, 83-B(5), 714–719. doi:10.1302/0301-620X.83B5.0830714

62 Roach, S. M., et al. (2015). "The impact of hip mobility on functional movement patterns in golfers." *Journal of Strength and Conditioning Research*, 29(7), 1865–1872. doi:10.1519/JSC.0000000000000835

63 Gellhorn, A. C., et al. (2013). "Osteoarthritis of the spine: The facet joints." *Nature Reviews Rheumatology*, 9(4), 216–224. doi:10.1038/nrrheum.2012.199

64 Hides, J. A., et al. (2011). "A clinical trial of motor control exercises for chronic low back pain." *Spine*, 36(5), 355–362. doi:10.1097/BRS.0b013e3181f9e8e0

65 Buckwalter, J. A., & Martin, J. A. (2004). "Sports and osteoarthritis." *Current Opinion in Rheumatology*, 16(5), 634–639. doi:10.1097/01.bor.0000132646.51326.39

66 Adams, M. A., & Roughley, P. J. (2006). "What is intervertebral disc degeneration, and what causes it?" *Spine*, 31(18), 2151–2161. doi:10.1097/01.brs.0000231761.73859.2c

67 Loeser, R. F., et al. (2012). "Osteoarthritis: A disease of the joint as an organ." *Arthritis & Rheumatism*, 64(6), 1697–1707. doi:10.1002/art.34453

68 Rajeswaran G, Turner M, Gissane C, Healy JC. MRI findings in the lumbar spines of asymptomatic elite junior tennis players. *Skeletal Radiol*. 2014 Jul;43(7):925-32. doi: 10.1007/s00256-014-1862-1. Epub 2014 Apr 2. PMID: 24691895

69 Mulvey, M. R., et al. (2013). "Modest association of joint hypermobility with disabling and limiting musculoskeletal pain: Results from a large-scale general population-based survey." *Arthritis Care & Research*, 65(8), 1325–1333. doi:10.1002/acr.21979

Chapter 6: Tune Me

1 https://www.learnreligions.com/six-blind-men-and-the-elephant-1770380

2 Black, P. H. (2002). "Stress and the inflammatory response: A review of neurogenic inflammation." *Brain, Behavior, and Immunity*, 16(6), 622–653. doi:10.1016/S0889-1591(02)00021-1

3 Kox, M., et al. (2014). "Voluntary activation of the sympathetic nervous system and attenuation of the innate immune response in humans." *Proceedings of the*

National Academy of Sciences, 111(20), 7379–7384. doi:10.1073/pnas.1322174111

4   Shaffer, F., & Ginsberg, J. P. (2017). "An overview of heart rate variability metrics and norms." *Frontiers in Public Health*, 5, 258. doi:10.3389/fpubh.2017.00258

5   Louw, A., et al. (2011). "The effect of neuroscience education on pain, disability, anxiety, and stress in chronic musculoskeletal pain." *Archives of Physical Medicine and Rehabilitation*, 92(12), 2041–2056. doi:10.1016/j.apmr.2011.07.198

6   Ehde, D. M., et al. (2014). "Cognitive-behavioral therapy for individuals with chronic pain: Efficacy, innovations, and directions for research." *American Psychologist*, 69(2), 153–166. doi:10.1037/a0035747

7   Tang, Y.-Y., Hölzel, B. K., & Posner, M. I. (2015). "The neuroscience of mindfulness meditation." *Nature Reviews Neuroscience*, 16(4), 213–225. doi:10.1038/nrn3916

8   Goyal, M., et al. (2014). "Meditation programs for psychological stress and well-being: A systematic review and meta-analysis." *JAMA Internal Medicine*, 174(3), 357–368. doi:10.1001/jamainternmed.2013.13018

9   Giugliano, D., et al. (2006). "The effects of diet on inflammation: Emphasis on the metabolic syndrome." *Journal of the American College of Cardiology*, 48(4), 677–685. doi:10.1016/j.jacc.2006.03.052

10 Casas, R., et al. (2014). "The effects of the Mediterranean diet on biomarkers of vascular wall inflammation and plaque vulnerability in subjects with coronary heart disease." *American Journal of Clinical Nutrition*, 99(6), 1419–1426. doi:10.3945/ajcn.113.080531

11 Irwin, M. R., et al. (2016). "Sleep disturbance, sleep duration, and inflammation: A systematic review and meta-analysis of cohort studies and experimental sleep deprivation." *Biological Psychiatry*, 80(1), 40–52. doi:10.1016/j.biopsych.2015.06.014

12 Hirshkowitz, M., et al. (2015). "National Sleep Foundation's sleep time duration recommendations: Methodology and results summary." *Sleep Health*, 1(1), 40–43. doi:10.1016/j.sleh.2014.12.010

13 Huberman Lab podcast episode 68 "Using Light (Sunlight, Blue Light & Red Light) to Optimize Health," April 18, 2022.

14 Opal, S. M., & DePalo, V. A. (2000). "Anti-inflammatory cytokines." *Chest*, 117(4), 1162–1172. doi:10.1378/chest.117.4.1162

15 Kiesel, K. B., et al. (2021). "Effects of multifidus-targeted neurostimulation on lumbar spine stability and pain in patients with chronic low back pain." *Spine*

Journal, 21(9), S45–S46. doi:10.1016/j.spinee.2021.05.116

16 McGill, S. M., et al. (2009). "Comparison of trunk muscle activity during simultaneous loading and dynamic movement: Implications for spine stability." *Journal of Electromyography and Kinesiology*, 19(2), e88–e96. doi:10.1016/j.jelekin.2007.10.007

17 Carey, D. G. (2009). "Quantifying differences in the 'fat burning' zone and the aerobic zone: Implications for training." *Journal of Strength and Conditioning Research*, 23(7), 2090–2095. doi:10.1519/JSC.0b013e3181bac5c5

18 Sahrmann, S. A. (2002). *Diagnosis and Treatment of Movement Impairment Syndromes*. Mosby. ISBN: 978-0801672057

19 Kendall, F. P., et al. (2005). *Muscles: Testing and Function, with Posture and Pain* (5th ed.). Lippincott Williams & Wilkins. ISBN: 978-0781747806

20 Janda, V. (1987). "Muscles and motor control in low back pain: Assessment and management." In *Physical Therapy of the Low Back* (pp. 253–278). Churchill Livingstone.

21 Hayden, J. A., et al. (2005). "Systematic review: Strategies for using exercise therapy to improve outcomes in chronic low back pain." *Annals of Internal Medicine*, 142(9), 776–785. doi:10.7326/0003-4819-142-9-200505030-00014

ILLUSTRATIONS

{ DR. SEAN WHEELER

Dr. Sean Wheeler has long been obsessed with pain. How pain and its absence, affects behavior, competitiveness, and quality of life.

This obsession turned passion sparked **a medical career investigating pain**, leading to a new way of understanding—and treating—back, neck and shoulder pain, to change the way musculoskeletal pain and injuries are treated—forever.

Having served as team physician for several member NCAA, NAIA, and NJCAA athletic programs, Dr. Sean is invited to speak at venues such as the University of Notre Dame Athletics Department.

Awarded a Doctor of Medicine from the University of Kansas School of Medicine, and board-certified in **Sports Medicine and Pain Management**, he has practiced medicine for 30 years. His passions remain Susie, his wife and their six children, playing guitar, and patients everywhere.

www.ingramcontent.com/pod-product-compliance
Lightning Source LLC
Chambersburg PA
CBHW070909130626
46555CB00001B/64